# THE REST OF THE TRUTH

## Second Edition:

Many Revisions Since 2009

Fast Weight Loss Programs/Bariatric Surgery

**Maintenance since 1996. No Boot Camps, no Cross Fit. Moderation leads to lifetime consistency!**

*by*

# Pamela Harrelson

Personal Trainer Since 1997

Nutrition Coach Under Umbrella of Registered Dieticians

American Council on Exercise

This message includes:

"Loving, Faith-Based Guidelines"

Copyright 2019 Pamela Harrelson,
All rights reserved.

Published in eBook format by eBookIt.com
http://www.eBookIt.com

ISBN-13: 978-1-4566-3402-5

No part of this book may be reproduced in any form or by any electronic or mechanical means including information storage and retrieval systems, without permission in writing from the author. The only exception is by a reviewer, who may quote short excerpts in a review.

*"Pam is a definite needed addition to obesity surgeries and rapid weight loss diets of various kinds. She picks up where the operation leaves off. She has a great personality, is easy to work with and has a tremendous passion to help us all. Her own story coincides with so many others. Saturday's workshop was great."*

Garie Friloux,
Gastric Bypass patient, Mandeville, LA.

*"Pam's message, combined with bariatric surgery, is what I have needed to reclaim my health and vitality. Pam has great passion to help bariatric patients toward lifetime weight maintenance. A significant number of us struggle to maintain, on one diet after another, and Pam's mission is to help us gain the balance we deserve after this ultimate decision."*

Dr. Catherine Hebert Carpenter
Mandeville, LA

# Disclaimer: This is not a diet book!

This book is not intended as a substitute for the medical advice of physicians. The reader should regularly consult a physician in matters relating to his/her health and particularly with respect to any symptoms that may require diagnosis or medical attention.

Pam Harrelson is neither a Bariatric nutrition expert nor a clinical nutrition expert. She is a certified Personal Trainer in athletic clubs and a certified nutrition consultant within those clubs, under the umbrella of Registered Dieticians only (not diet doctors.) She simply shares her own "tweaks" in nutrition that have delivered her from food addiction, based on her own personality. She refers you to websites in her appendix who are professional experts!

# Table of Contents

INTRODUCTION ................................................................. 4
ACKNOWLEDGEMENTS ................................................... 6
DEDICATED TO MY HUSBAND OF 30 YEARS! ........... 8
CHAPTER ONE ................................................................. 18
    OUR MEMOIR: WHERE WAS THE TRUTH? ................ 18
    GOOD ADVICE FROM A THERAPIST ON BODY IMAGE AFTER A LARGE WEIGHT LOSS. ............................... 33
CHAPTER TWO ................................................................ 38
    THE TRUTH WILL SET YOU FREE BUT FIRST IT WILL MAKE YOU MISERABLE! ................................................ 38
    Section One: God's "permissive will" and God's "perfect will." ............................................................................. 38
    Section Two: Moving on ............................................. 41
    Section Three: Let's move forward psychologically and spiritually. ................................................................. 47
    Section Four: Our hearts have to change first ............ 48
    Section Five: What's controlling your mind? ............ 51
    Section Six: The four P's: Prayer, Preparation, Planning, and Patience ................................................................ 54
    Section Seven: SUPERNATURAL OPPOSITION must be overcome with SUPERNATURAL MEANS ................. 55
CHAPTER THREE ............................................................. 64
    METABOLISM AND GENETICS ................................. 64
    Nutshell Study: Moseby Yearbook January, 1998 ....... 66
    PROTEIN REQUIREMENTS: (BY REGISTERED DIETICIANS WHO STUDY NUTRITION FOR YEARS) .. 75
    Genetic Make-up ........................................................ 78

| CHAPTER FOUR | 88 |
| --- | --- |
| KEYWORDS FOR CHANGE | 88 |
| The mind can be changed! | 88 |
| IMPATIENCE "WAITING, WAITING, WAITING" | 94 |
| **CHAPTER FIVE** | **112** |
| DISCOVER A LOVE FOR MOVEMENT AT ANY AGE! | 112 |
| **CHAPTER SIX** | **128** |
| PERSONAL TRAINING FROM MY PERSPECTIVE | 128 |
| **CHAPTER SEVEN** | **146** |
| FIND A "PAM'S BULLET" THAT MAY BE LIFE CHANGING. | 146 |
| **CHAPTER EIGHT** | **166** |
| IMPORTANT UPDATE ON PAM AT AGE 69 (THE BULK OF THIS MANUSCRIPT WAS WRITTEN AT AGE 58) | 166 |
| **CHAPTER NINE** | **178** |
| REDEEMED BY GOD'S GRACE. LET GOD WRITE HIS STORY INTO OURS! | 178 |
| Appendix | 200 |
| A brief list of more structured help for you in the form of websites and books. | 200 |
| **NOTES** | **204** |

# INTRODUCTION

*Lifetime weight maintenance starts with the mind, not with a diet, and certainly not with a scalpel on the operating table.*

*If you are obese, pre-bariatric surgery, post-bariatric surgery, or even just an average-sized person caught for decades in the terrible cycle of dieting, deprivation; a feeling of "food addiction," I believe there are bound to be some life changing points for you somewhere in this manuscript. This would be for bariatric surgery patients or for <u>anyone</u> on the miserable dieting roller coaster. I have not been on a diet since 1996! Set FREE! A process of full deliverance that can happen for you! My surgery does NOT prevent me from gaining weight….. my brain does! This is evident from the vast number of bariatric patients who regain weight.*

I have been pleased at more stories of Bariatric Surgery patients maintaining weight permanently since these surgeries started decades ago. However, I am **shocked** in 2020 at the substantial number of them who regain a lot of weight or all their weight after 5 years. I have discovered this fact while working at a large athletic club once again and having many consults. **The surgeons operate on our stomachs, not our brains!**

My story and suggestions reveal the convictions that God can lead one to in following solid Biblical principles, but also reveals that a feeling of **condemnation is never from God.** Too many of us who love the Lord find ourselves in this struggle to make changes from an addictive, emotionally-obsessive rut to a system of self-control that is **not** reliant solely on will-power.

God's amazing interventions in my obesity struggle demonstrate His gentle and *total understanding* of our human weakness. It expresses a profound belief that with reliance on our faith, a strong relationship with God, and the guidance of Biblical scripture, our faith can then translate to more self-control and motivation in the areas of nutrition and exercise. I pray to expedite this process for you! God is **for you** and wants you to get to the other side of this issue to have the energy you need for others. I did after 38 years! (from age 8)

# We can live life to the fullest, enslaved to nothing!

# ACKNOWLEDGEMENTS

Thank you to my children who have allowed me to share our personal story because they know it will help others.

Thanks to the Southern Christian Writer's Guild who have supported me and encouraged me in this message.

Thank you to Personal Training clients. Mary, Kim, Danielle, Julia, and Sandy who were willing to take the time to read this and encourage me that it was "important" and worth the sacrifice of 2 ½ years.

Thanks to Maureen Eames who has been a reader with sweet reviews and forewords on a previous book. She is also a lifetime maintenance story.

Thank you to Lynda Deal, who encouraged me immensely from the beginning to the very end, while she persevered in her own lifelong dream. Lynda, we did not give up.

Thank you to Debbie Barr, author of "Children of Divorce" and "Keeping Love Alive as Memories Fade" (about Alzheimer's) for all the advice about the publishing world, and sending some research.

Thanks to Ruth Gilly Kenyan in Texas for being one of my readers of all my books with wonderful reviews. She was a "target reader" in my mind. A person not known to me from the great state of Texas! She is the most encouraging person to me in my attempt to help other patients. She is an inspiration to others in her lifetime weight maintenance, finally after two surgeries (like me).

Thanks to Rich Sousa, in Oregon, who fully supported me and encouraged me. That was quite a compliment since he is a very critical personality and a real thinker. He was 100% for all of it!

Thank you to Tracy Asmussen, my youngest sister. She is the *only* person who has spent literally *hundreds* of hours helping me to clarify my message. She did this while she was in the middle of all the red tape in international travels, taking care of a sick child, getting one daughter into college, getting ready for a visit from one son in the military, and her volunteer work with a children's home. She spent massive hours helping me to clarify 49,000 words of content.

This message *would not be in print to help the obese and those who love them* without my sister's love and passion for others. She "pulled" the various messages out of me, through much weeping and hard work! Though her own fitness level is nearly perfect, she had a full and intuitive understanding of who I wanted to help and why. I admire her intelligence and writing talents. I don't have a writer's talent, but just an important message that she understood. I am still in disbelief at her unending hours of work with attachments back and forth from Bolivia, South America. She continually refused financial compensation. *My never ending love and thanks to Tracy Asmussen, my precious little sister.*

# DEDICATED TO MY HUSBAND OF 30 YEARS!

*Robert Al Harrelson July 15, 1947– July 9, 2000*
### Dozens of unhealthy diets
### Two Bariatric Surgeries

This is an e-mail that Al wrote to a friend before he died in 2000. She sent it to me in the regular mail just two days after his funeral. We had never met her. They were each involved in Harrelson genealogy research online. You will be able to see from his letter to Dee that he wanted our book written. It delighted me and surprised me when I read his thoughts to a stranger. He also called me his "lovely wife!" In it he confirms our suffering over the years. Al's words in this e-mail reminded me of *many conversations that he and I had* about **believing in me** to write this book in order to help others in bondage to this terrible addiction. Al died three years after his gastric by-pass surgery.

*From: AL H To: Dee*

*Date: Monday, March 13, 2000 Subject: Prospect Concern*

*Hi Dee,*

*"As for me, as you can read in my link, I am waiting on a heart transplant. By the grace of God I have been able to stay at home most of the time. Since I can rest and*

*take my medication I have been able to have a quality life style. As for my possible surgery, recent tests in the last 2 weeks indicate I need another angiogram tomorrow - to determine if I need bypass surgery. My cardiologist believes it will be necessary, however, we shall see tomorrow. My diagnosis has been dilated cardiomyopathy with an ejection fraction as low as 114k.*

*Am I concerned with the prospect of surgery? For years I had the Type A lifestyle. The first time I was diagnosed with DCM in 1986, I took my office to the hospital with me. In 1996 I had another major episode with DCM. My cardiologist told me I needed to retire from work. You know how we Type A's are (in one category), we go through a stage of denial. I loved my job more than I loved my family and God. In 1997, God put me flat on my back again. I realized then I could not keep up with the job. My decision after much prayer was to have a closer relationship with God and not worry about the future. Since retiring I do not worry about things. My family knows where I stand.*

*Almost everything is done in my life, except knowing the last thing I am expected to do. My children know that if I am called to leave this earth they have a father that loves them with all my heart, despite how sick it is. They know that I now set the example God wanted me to leave them with.*

*The same for my lovely wife, Pam. She raised our children and now she has finally started her career as a Personal Trainer where she can help others. She hopes one day to write a book about our experiences with obesity, bariatric surgery, and what needs to be done to change a person's life style before it has been ruined as mine was. Hopefully she will be able to do this using my life's example and her life's example. She has changed her presentation title from "The Dieting Mentality" to "Where's the Truth?"*

*Thanks for all your effort on the NCBLAOEN list. I plan on emailing you again soon!"*

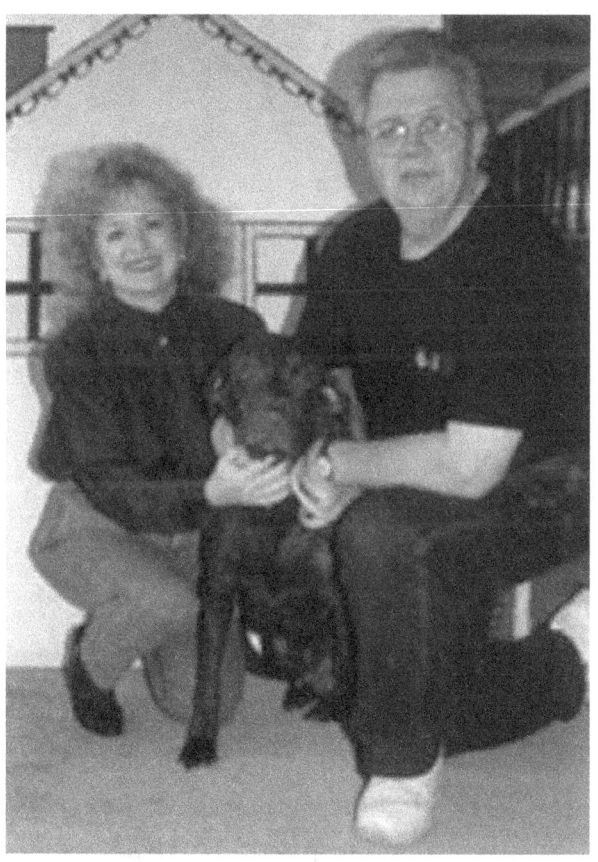

His weight was down in this picture but his heart was already ruined from years of obesity and poor genetics. He said almost everything in his life is done, except knowing the **last** thing he is supposed to do. The moment I read the letter, standing by my mailbox, I knew that it was a message from his grave. What was the last thing he was supposed to do? Could it be inspiring me through this surprise email, delivered to me through a stranger?

**Dedication to Al continued, including our radical diets.**

There were so many fast weight loss diets; I think we did them all. The doctors were there to "serve our impatience" and as far as I can see, overweight **Americans still want a fast fix.**

Briefly, I will share with you that we were *each from slender families*, which included our parents and siblings. This is worth mentioning, because so many stories we hear are about the entire family overeating and everyone in the obese category. I was on a strict diet from age seven, which maintained a slender size for me 95% of the time. The doctors prescribed strong amphetamines for me starting at age ten. I "flew" around on the playground, "speeded" up, but I stayed slim, like the rest of my family. However, all of this effort created life-long food disorders and contributed to many other problems growing up. Food should never be presented to a child as an issue in their growing up years. I feel my mom and I were victims of the new dieting mentality in the 1950's and 60's. Al was on the obese side since age eight, because he was raised in a "working poor" family, and he was not allowed outside to play while his parents worked. He overate in quantities while sitting and watching TV.

In contrast to me, he developed a very balanced, likable personality. My food disorder, a very low thyroid as a child which creates depression, and the amphetamines, I believe all contributed to create many psychological problems as I developed, which God has resolved over the years.

I really can't remember the names of all of our diets which started in 1971 as a couple. I know that there were many which were liquid-based, where we could eat anything we wanted for supper after fasting on liquid concoctions all day. Al always lost his weight very, very fast on these diets, but he also always gained it back very fast, which was not healthy. I lost slowly because short folks have a slower basal metabolic rate, and even more so with no exercise, as was my case.

On one of the liquid fasts which Al had been on for three months, he developed a serious bowel impaction. I will never forget it because he was rushed to the emergency room for help in passing it. It was a high protein diet and there was just not enough fiber in it to keep his bowels moving, along with a sedentary lifestyle.

We went on the Dr. Atkins program as soon as it came out, after the birth of our first child in 1973. I remember the little "ketosis" sticks we used and the cravings I had for "green peas." Psychologically, if a food was forbidden, we craved it. We almost always went crazy when we finished a diet, eating whatever we had been denied during that time, thus gaining weight back quickly. We used the Atkins diet **often** because it "worked every time!"

Al never liked the diet pills. I continued to use those from time to time and basically I was a speed freak whenever I was on them. We also tried the non-medical approaches, which were the crazy little diet plans people passed around in the office. Among these were the "cabbage diet" and the "ice cream diet!" They always introduced the diets by saying, "It works!" I now know when someone says "it works," he is talking about fast weight-loss. We latched onto that promise with hope, while **maintenance remained an afterthought** we just didn't want to take the time to think about. Actually, I don't believe we thought that anyone ever maintained a weight loss. We just thought that one was on a diet or one was gaining weight. It seems as if we became so overwhelmed with the hope for dramatic weight loss at hand, that any thought of how to maintain that for the long-term wasn't considered important at the time.

This cycle went on as a couple for twenty-four years! The diet "works?" Well, it works all 150 times! The *way we lose the weight* makes a huge difference in being able to maintain it without an impossible struggle.

> *Prohibiting foods or making them forbidden reinforces the fear that food is dangerous and cannot be handled. To create an entire weight-loss plan based on this assumption is both unfair and unnecessary. In addition, when certain foods are characterized as "forbidden" they can become more desirable and harder to eat in moderate amounts. What is*

> more realistic is to encourage eating of moderate amounts of a wide variety of tasty, nutritious, and satisfying foods.1

Eventually, we did become disgusted with a life of unbalanced nutrition; in essence, two weeks of cabbage, or two weeks of ice cream. Then we heard about Weight Watchers. Back then they did the "food exchanges" which is basically the same concept Registered Dieticians teach on the food pyramid, with some caloric formulas from textbooks. Weight Watchers taught the "truth" and still does.

Our weight loss on their program, however, was very slow and did not satisfy our impatience. I realize now that the right amount of calories, which Weight Watchers provides, also requires a walking program if you want to lose weight consistently enough to provide encouragement. You don't feel deprived or hungry on a program like this so you can keep going long term, if you are patient. The payoff is that your metabolism also "grows" in the right direction. However, at the time we used the program, the exercise part was not as emphasized as it is now. I recommend their program over most others, as long as you obey their walking program that they more avidly promote now.

The textbook formula on correct weight-loss calories for me is 1,200 a day.

I am only five feet tall (barely) so this is not the same formula as for those who are taller. On Weight Watchers, I lost the first two weeks and felt full and satisfied on their choices

---

[1] Ronna Kabtznic PHD in Nutrition

and treats. If I had only walked, (as I finally did in 1995), I would have continued to lose consistently on the 1,200 calories until the weight was off. At that time, Al and I did not "believe" in exercise. We only believed in dieting.

If I had understood that I would lose weight slowly walking forty minutes, five days weekly, while eating 1,200 calories, and that it would have been accomplished in eighteen months, I never would have had this surgery. If you know your nutritional values you can have a lot of food on 1,200 calories. **Later, because I did not diet below 1200 and hurt my metabolism, I got to have 1800 calories per day.**

We lived together like this for 24 long years, losing and gaining, losing and gaining large amounts of weight. Maintenance was something that never occurred to us. We just did not believe that such a "third category" existed. We saw people who always maintained their weight, but we thought that was just "lucky genetics". We never noticed that they *filled up* on lower calorie items, still enjoyed richer foods in smaller portions, and were walkers. We were still in denial.

Al's favorite diet doctor was a local. He was an internist and a surgeon and had a flourishing local business using liquid diets for fast weight-loss. He encouraged his patients to lose as fast as they could. He had always been very fit himself and loved strict eating. He was also an avid exerciser.

We went to him repeatedly because his method "worked every time." He always told us it was alright to fail and start over. The program was expensive and our insurance paid for part of it. This doctor did recommend moderate, regular exercise: however, he approved of Al running! This is not something that I would ever recommend for a heavy person. Someone using this type of exercise strictly for weight loss, even though he may like it for a while, will likely not going to keep doing it for a lifetime. A "runner is a runner is a runner." We were not runners. A good lifetime walking program is what should have been encouraged for people like us who had never practiced a rigorous exercise program before. Also, on a very low calorie diet combined with running, your metabolism is even more decreased.

We_turned to radical diets as a means of weight loss and followed the "herd" like lame sheep. Registered Dietitians, (who I only pay attention to now) focus on healthy, delicious food. They do not condone the diet doctors in regard to extreme diets. Registered Dieticians have Master's and/or a PHD Degree in Nutrition. Diet doctors do not. Bariatric physicians have changed everything about nutrition since they design different plumbing for our bodies. I still pay more attention to Registered Dieticians. They have not disappointed me.

To me, food is fuel but it should also be enjoyed. We never enjoyed the ketosis plans but repeated them over and over. A diet where we stay in "ketosis" is creating a chemical imbalance. Ugh!

To maintain ketosis, you must continue to eat a very low-carb diet. It's a plan that you must stick to without fail. I have learned since 1996 the enjoyment of the 80/20 process. 80%

good and 20% bad using the wide variety of foods that God has planned for us.

A ketosis plan for folks who need a "cheat" day left Al and I feeling that we had axe murdered our parents! We had to start from scratch again to get back into ketosis, which took a few days or weeks.

With all the side effects and complications this ketosis plan has, I'm truly surprised by the popularity it has re-gained in 2019. It is not enjoyable. We never enjoyed it. Always felt deprived.

In my book I will describe what pleasant boundaries are for myself and many others. My Mom was never overweight. She was never on any of these radical diet plans. She ate a wide variety of foods with portion control in the richer items. This is enjoyment of God's creation and much healthier in dozens of ways.

# CHAPTER ONE

## *OUR MEMOIR: WHERE WAS THE TRUTH?*

When my husband and I had the new gastric by-pass surgery in 1995 and in 1996, we were like all potential patients. We had suffered despair, failures, and hopelessness undergoing strict diets and previous obesity surgeries for twenty-four years as a couple. I had been on this maddening roller coaster since age seven or eight! We trusted all the doctors who wrote the fast weight-loss books and the local diet physicians. Of course we trusted them; they were doctors!

We had great hope that the brand new surgery, which was about four years old, would make our dreams come true. Our dream was no more dieting, no more gaining and losing, rather a permanent and lasting weight loss to be achieved with great ease through surgery alone. We prayed to be released from our deep mental bondage through "physician-assisted starvation"[2] forever. It appeared that perhaps this surgery was finally the miracle cure, as long as you obeyed instructions while it healed.

---

[2] *Losing It*, by Laura Fraser, by Random House, 1995

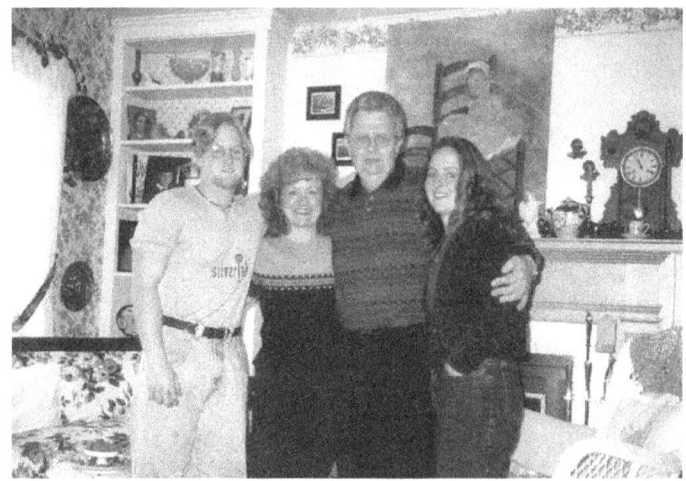

*Pictured is our family in 1997. My husband, Al, passed away in July of 2000 of obesity related heart failure and diabetes. His weight was way down in this picture. I was just beginning weight maintenance after losing 96 pounds slowly in 18 months (an average of 5.5 pounds per month)*

In 1996, only four months post-op from the obesity surgery, I realized that I was in the deepest emotional pit I had *ever been* in concerning weight-loss failure. I had come to realize, that very week, that I could out eat the surgery with no problem at all. I had lost 37 pounds just from the required fasting after the surgery, as well as being very sick from the actual surgery. (They had no laparoscopic procedure at that time and being cut wide open was of course a huge trauma to the body).

Of course I had lost the same 37 pounds many times over 24 years. I always regained it because I depended on low calorie, fast weight-loss diets alone and did not exercise consistently, if at all. These practices slow down the metabolic rate, as fully documented in Chapter Three. This truth is biologically sound and the way that God made our bodies to protect us in times of famine. The puzzling truth is that few physicians, even weight-loss physicians, warn patients about this. They simply tell us what we want to hear, that fast weight loss "works." It is a "revolving door" mentality.

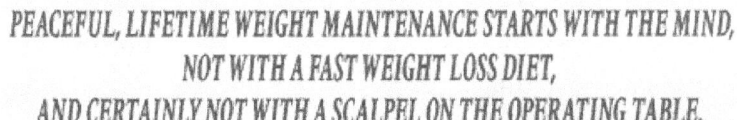

PEACEFUL, LIFETIME WEIGHT MAINTENANCE STARTS WITH THE MIND, NOT WITH A FAST WEIGHT LOSS DIET, AND CERTAINLY NOT WITH A SCALPEL ON THE OPERATING TABLE.

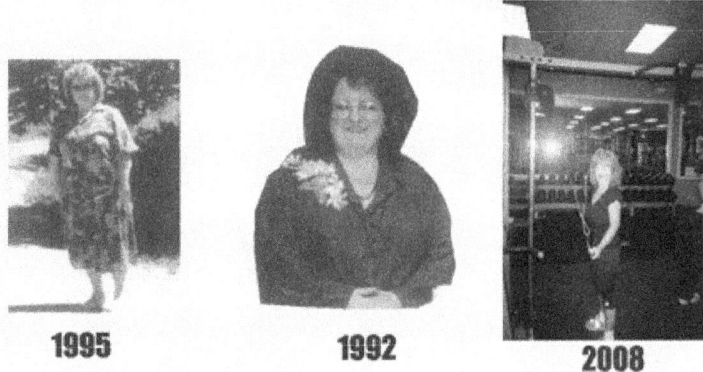

**1995**      **1992**      **2008**

Sixteen years earlier was one year after our gastric-stapling surgeries. An outright miracle was marketed, as it always is with a new surgery. I had practiced a great deal of denial in that year regarding what was happening with the effectiveness of the surgery.

As a result, I regained all of 100 pounds I had lost in the next four years. (Al's surgery staples broke loose in a few months and he had followed all instructions as well). I became very depressed and confused about why I regained half of the weight back on a strict 1,000 calories a day. There was nothing in *popular print* at that time about metabolism shutting down through starvation (I had lost the weight on a mere 600 calories a day). No one believed me when I told them I was gaining weight back on a mere 1,000 calories, but this was absolutely true! That was one thing I was not in denial about. At the time, all I knew about calories was the starvation calorie amount on the one hand, and that I had originally become obese from binging, that is, consuming enormous amounts of calories in one sitting. When I became obese again four years after the gastric-stapling, I no longer had a binging problem, but *snacked* all the time and never exercised.

I wanted to be able to face the truth this time around about the realistic effectiveness of the new gastric by-pass. I wanted to avoid the awful depression, in the event that this surgery was not a miracle either. Surgery failures have a high depression and suicide rate, according to one book written years ago as well as more *recent research.*[3] My personal opinion is that we do not have all the numbers because people are ashamed and the statistics are, therefore, most likely under-reported.

One night 4 months after the surgery in 1996, walking alone in my suburban neighborhood, I was still in great shock over the realizations of the gastric-bypass surgery. I had just discovered that I could eat more than the caloric amount needed to lose the weight! I was in no dangerous denial this time around (as I had been in 1981 after my first surgery), but *tremendous shock and fear gripped me.* I wanted to disappear into the woods as I walked that night. I hoped that a car or truck might hit me and put an end to it all. I did not know how I would face failure again if I couldn't lose the rest of the weight, or even worse, if I regained all that I had lost. I did not

---

[3] Losing It, Laura Fraser, Random House 1995

know how I would "save face" in the light of how the surgery was *continually advertised as impossible to regain weight*. If you couldn't lose weight after having your stomach stapled and your intestine altered, you must really be pathetic! People I loved would lose respect for me now more than ever. My husband's surgery was scheduled soon and he was full of hope. I absolutely could not tell him what I was experiencing. He had an obesity-related heart condition and needed to lose 125 pounds quickly or his life would be in imminent danger. I knew that Al would not exercise at all or at least not for long, as that had always been our shared lifestyle. I knew from experience that he lost weight very rapidly on fast weight loss procedures and that he was actually facing death this time with a bad heart, so I had to keep all the perplexing realizations to myself and not even tell the doctor. I hoped for the best with Al. Besides, I thought, maybe his outcome would be far different from my own. He was not a snacker but ate large meals, which exceeded his calorie boundaries.

As far as I knew, none of the surgeons or patients at that time were aware of the enlarged stoma problem, although it probably happened to others as well, despite the fact that they followed all the post-op instructions. *I felt entirely alone.* My body was mutilated inside with "new plumbing". The surgery was like being hit by a car and the recovery was terrible at that time.

I am sorry to be so dramatic, but on my walk that night, as I prayed and cried, I felt like a soldier facing death in a foxhole. This is where God climbed into that very, very deep foxhole with me. Somehow on that night, he gave me the courage to climb out, like a very brave warrior under fire. I had to be brave for my husband; I had to be totally silent about my fears. Once again, I was all alone in my knowledge of the surgery experience and **remained totally alone with it for** *years*. There was **no blogging on websites from other patients at that time. We could not compare notes.** Surgeons did not follow up with their patients for years as they do now. It seemed to me that everyone else in the clinic that had the surgery could hardly eat at all and lost 100 pounds in 4-8 months with great ease. They also lost their hair though, and I truly believe that my slow weight loss protected my hair! I was "shamed into silence"iiii; deathly afraid for Al. I wonder how many patients, over the years, have also been shamed into silence or committed suicide. We simply don't know. What I do know, is that while the regain is not entirely their fault, they are allowed to take all the blame while the medical community remains anywhere from vague to silent. This is, of course, my opinion based solely on personal experience and other people's testimonials also.

As I continued to walk slowly at night, and mulled over this situation, God used this deepest pit and foxhole to cut through all the brainwashing by different diet doctors that I had undergone and accepted for over thirty-five years, since age seven actually.

As I walked and prayed, I gained the courage (not knowing or understanding the future) to open my mind. My mind became wide open to information *other* than fast weight loss. I yearned for the whole truth and I embraced the truth for the first time in my whole life. This was because, in that deep pit, I let go of all denial, all fear, and especially, **all impatience** and I was open in my mind to embrace God's truth!

**Finally, after years of extreme measures, I came to "the end" of myself, and had to rely on the grace of God. When we use God's grace, He changes us little by little, in a long process where we become anchored and free forever.**

A short while later while employed at a medical university for doctors, nurses, and registered dieticians, I learned about eating six times a day and tracking the right amount of calories within my boundaries. I had never in my life *stayed* with a walking program so I had no idea yet how it would affect my body; therefore, I only prayed that I would maintain my present weight loss of 37 pounds! Never, ever did I think that I would continue to lose, moderately, slowly, and consistently! I was surprised each week when I did, in fact, do just that.

The malabsorption of calories and severe diarrhea that are often a result of the surgery tapered off within four months; years later my vitamin and mineral profile, including my B-12, is very good. I no longer need higher amounts of protein, and eat according to the "Choosemyplate" government guidelines with ease. My health profile (cholesterol, blood pressure, triglycerides, etc.) is like a twenty-five year-old's even without the high protein diet that is continually promoted with post-op patients. A high protein, low carb food program would seem like a *lifelong diet* for me, and I believe that the mentality of "low-carb, high-protein" pushed on post-op patients actually works against many of them by making them feel continually deprived. As a formerly obese person, I know the mentality, and I know exactly where "deprivation" leads. This is my personal opinion.

It no longer mattered that the weight loss was slow or when at regular intervals I reached a plateau and stopped losing weight for no good reason. God was ready to teach an open mind which was not saturated with impatience. I could now listen to the truth as it was gradually revealed to me. I had prayed for answers for years, but had not "listened" to God when I prayed. I wanted results very fast. I did not want to "learn" anything. Now, I was **ready to listen and accept any hard** work God had for me to do! *Therefore, many "divine interventions" began to occur in my life.*

**A DIVINE INTERVENTION:** When I was assigned by the state Civil Service to work as a secretary for a physician in the medical university, the first day was an amazing act of God. I could have been assigned to anyone. On my first day of work, as I slowly walked the hallways looking for the name of my **assigned doctor** on a door, I was **stunned when I finally found it and read the department name above it: "Nutrition and Metabolism."** The sixty-five year-old man behind the door turned out to be a world-renowned medical expert and professor (MD, PHD) on this topic. His assistant professor was also a registered dietician with a Master's degree. They were NOT diet doctors! They were strictly academic in teaching college students the truth about our bodies… and the truth does not change! I immediately felt that I had been brought to this office by God Himself, although I wasn't yet sure why.

Shortly after I began working in the doctor's office, I was amused by one file the doctor had that was nearly 40 years old. It was labeled "Fads." As I remember, unless the nutrition program I was asked to file was in accordance with the Food Pyramid or the Mediterranean Diet, it did not matter which famous diet doctor had written it, I was told to file it away in the "Fad" file. (I had done all those fads in the file myself!)

In my spare time I devoured textbook information on such topics as the "Law of Thermodynamics," basal metabolism, the Mosby Yearbook, all the basic caloric formulas, and the USDA food plate guidelines. I learned, among many other things, the reason why we require the right caloric amount when dieting, and the body's biological need for the **correct balance** of complex carbohydrates, protein, and fat. Also, there was much textbook information on exercise and how it raised metabolism, as long as you did not overdo it and the calories you consumed were not too low.

**I would never have lost such a great percentage of my excess weight or maintained my weight, even with the surgery, had God not placed me in this office. I firmly believe that God would not have blessed me in this center of education had I not finally embraced the fruit of the spirit patience, which pried opened my mind to the <u>truth</u>.**

This educational center showed me the truth of how God designed our bodies in regard to our wonderful metabolic thermostat. **(Excerpts in Chapter Three and resources listed on my Resource Page are from more academic experts than me in this field and they support my statements.** (Are you willing to open your mind to the truth that we still have by studying, as I finally did?) Why is it the truth? There are no ulterior motives from this academic group. These are Federal studies with *no financial gain*. This is an academic study taught to college students in the field of Nutrition and Metabolism. Long term studies, ongoing by Federal government, are not influenced by popular fads and diet doctors who make a fortune in fast weight loss. The studies are not influenced by slick marketing campaigns which promote foods as magic or evil. These things all fade away—always! Those people do not care about balance. They just want to give the public what they want and it is a trillion dollar industry. I experienced the lies firsthand for 35 years.

Daily I devoured these truths and other morsels of information which fed my spirit and soul. As a result, I soon incorporated exercise into my lunch break. I made a deal with the doctor by offering to stay 30 minutes later if he could give me a longer lunch break for this purpose and to my delight, he agreed. I lost the rest of the weight while working for him. The associate professor offered to analyze my food records and declared them to be balanced, according to the food pyramid guidelines. (The food pyramid is now "Choosemyplate" and is on the resource page.) I used the calorie formulas found in the textbooks, (which, compared to my past experience with dieting, were relatively high) and consistently walked forty minutes, five days each week. I lost an average of five- and-a-half pounds per month. There was no counting carbs, as the post-op patients do presently. (I only did very high protein during the first four months so that I would not lose my hair.)

I stayed away from foods that made me sick, as a result of the by-pass, but consumed many healthy foods and some treats. I could eat fattening chocolate candy as long as it had plenty of fat in it which metabolized the sugar. This prevented the painful stomach aches (dumping) I had been promised with the surgery, if I ate sweets. However, sweets that contained no fat did cause dumping (like sweet tea and hard candy.) I could still eat my favorite Reese Cup which I refrained from as much as possible. However, I treat myself on a regular basis to "forbidden" foods, in order not to have a deprivation mentality backfire on me and then use snacking to address stress.

**I became quite satisfied to lose slowly on the "greatest amount of food with the least amount of exercise"** (Apex Fitness quote; I was certified by Apex fitness group in 1999.) As I said in my outline, I lost 96 pounds in eighteen months, not in *eight* months as most patients my size do. I went from 211 pounds, at five feet tall, to 115 pounds at age forty-six. After I started weight lifting at age forty-seven, I gained about five pounds of lean body mass, but was smaller around! This muscle provided more calories for me "at rest" also!

**As I studied metabolism facts, I slowly realized that I was not one of the unlucky patients because mine was not a super-fast weight loss; rather, I was one of the very fortunate because my weight loss was gradual over a longer period of time. This method raised my basal metabolism, making weight maintenance easier and allowing many more calories. Therefore I am not complaining about the stoma stretching early. I am quite happy that God allowed this to happen. His**

plan was different than my own. I have not been on a weight loss diet in 24 years! I have not fallen off this "easy wagon" once! Age has changed some things though. Thank God I had "room" for a little old age spread after Menopause and my spinal injury (see Chapter Eight).

I did not know it way back in 1996, but as I faced maintenance, *my metabolism was about to soar*. One year later, I could maintain 120 pounds by eating 1,800 calories a day and exercising only four hours a week, which included weight-lifting and 5 – 35 minute jogs per week. Very lifetime program!

I never overdid the exercise, risking injury or burnout. I always looked forward to my time alone during walks, (later jogs), with the wind in my hair and the sun in my face. Twenty four years later, I *still feel the same!* I have not been on a strict diet once since 1996 (I methodically **raised** my calories at that time to begin maintaining). I truly wish the same for all people stuck on a dieting roller-coaster of any kind, **even the person with just a recurrent ten pound problem**. I had those people coming into my Personal Training office quite frequently! They are also burned out on the endless cycle of gaining, losing and re-gaining. Nothing is more discouraging for anyone than a sense of repeated failure, and this often leads to poor decisions full of desperation.

**DIVINE INTERVENTION**: Before I resigned from the physician's office, I had a goal to help my son attain his Personal Trainer's Certification. He loved the gym and I knew this was something he was interested in. We each ordered all the study materials and I read them carefully in order to coach him for the impending three-day-course and exam for the "Beginner's Certification." We drove out of town and attended the course together which was taught by two exercise physiologists from Boston, Massachusetts. I had no intention of becoming a personal trainer myself! I had only wanted to help my son who needed a little extra motivating in his life, because he was still in his teen-age years and needed a little push. However, I came back with a certificate, hung up a flyer to help people at my home, and soon began to see three clients a week doing a walking program! At that point in time I could not have anticipated the vast amount of experience I would eventually gain working in athletic clubs or the certificates I would continue to add to my portfolio. With my personal history of dieting and obesity, this would have seemed too surreal! Even today, it still seems miraculous to me. I became a noted trainer for years, helping many people! This was after years of food addiction and no consistent exercise.

**DIVINE INTERVENTION**: At the time that Al became disabled by heart disease and had to quit his job, there was a large athletic club located in our neighborhood. I had always been too ashamed to even go in there, thinking it was only for the ultra-fit! However, when I got the nerve to approach them and told them I had a Personal Training Certification and three successful home clients, they **actually** hired me! With my *pathetic background, I simply could not believe it*, as this was a very progressive athletic club. I continued to study all textbook and personal training information I could get my hands on while working with many clients during a fifty-hour work week. Since I am not an aerobics instructor, I have never exercised with my PT clients. Like everyone else, I had to do my work out on my own, but the club, of course, gave me easy access to this.

**DIVINE INTERVENTION**: The owner of the club, where I worked, due to his own weight struggle, looked far and wide for the right company to turn his certified Personal Trainers at the club into "weight-loss pros" instead of just weight-lifting experts. The company he hired was called Apex Fitness Group, out of California. There was no other club for hundreds of miles around that paid the

$50,000 fee for this company. Many of their employees were former competitive body-builders, but most of them had their Master's degrees in Exercise Physiology and some were even Registered Dieticians.

While attending their classes and all of their quarterly training meetings, I was stunned once again. **The material was exactly the same material I had seen in the physician's office at the medical school. My physician's name (my former employer) was even in listed in one of their many medical biographies**. There were only a handful of clubs in this part of the South where certified trainers were under the Apex "umbrella" of Registered Dieticians and Exercise Physiologists. Under God's umbrella and design for my life, I landed in one of them! God continued to "underline" the truth for me with miraculous interventions. **I express these truths with utter confidence. The truth of how God made us has always been here and documented, but is distorted or** hidden by our impatience and the greed of others taking advantage of our desperation.

**I lost the weight on the "greatest amount of food with the least amount of exercise." My metabolism soared and maintenance has been easy with a lot of calories and a consistent, moderate exercise plan. Many post-op patients are still on miserable diets.** This does not have to be the case. I maintain my small size by "eating and moving." I don't diet and don't count carbs, which is nothing but another diet. I eat a balanced diet and keep an eye on calories. I am able to have a proper, liberal amount of calories (based on physics formulas listed Chapter Three). I am grateful for the edge that the surgery still gives me in some respects. The pouch is still strong. However, I can eat large enough meals and snack the wrong snacks to have far more than my calorie boundaries require for this short height and BMI guideline.

I am grateful that my stoma stretched prematurely because this resulted in hard work on my part, which resulted in a strong metabolism. I raised my metabolism on a slow weight loss regimen with higher calories, with regular but moderate exercise. The bariatric clinics **promote the promise** of malabsorption of calories to desperate people. I know that there is malabsorption of minerals and vitamins because I have to take iron for anemia despite the fact that I eat a very nutritious balance of carbohydrates, fat, and protein. Despite the fact that I lift weights and have an active lifestyle, I just developed osteoporosis in 2013 (bone loss) which is cited as a potential health risk for patients. My vitamin B-12, however, remains high with a small supplement tablet.

**I gain weight on an intake of calories that exceeds my formula requirements, just as <u>any other</u> person would do and as many post-op patients do**. I lost my weight slowly on 1200 calories daily with 4 hours of consistent exercise per week. This *matched up* to my academic formulas (Chapter Three tells you how to do the formula). This truth is evidenced by the many who are on the various surgery blogging web sites and they are struggling post-op not to regain their weight. In fact, one of my **physicians, a well-educated surgeon**, recently gained twenty-five pounds back at the **beginning of her second year post-op.** This was with the *inability to binge*, but only because of *snacking and not exercising*. Malabsorption of calories? In 2020 I personally know a number of patients who have regained all their weight after the Sleeve surgery. BEWARE of this marketing tool! LEARN facts and start habits to help you during your "4 year window of ease" after the surgery! That window of ease is your miracle, short of moving to a third world country for 2 years!

## *GOOD ADVICE FROM A THERAPIST ON BODY IMAGE AFTER A LARGE WEIGHT LOSS.*

This is a very brief testimonial on my personal experience with body image, which I hope will be valuable to those who have had a large weight loss and are troubled in some ways as they cope with their new image. Although my book's focus is on health, the negative side of fast weight loss, and not on how we look, body image is everywhere in our culture, and it can "take over" if we are not cautious!

In late 1996, I was still working at the medical school during the very initial phase of weight maintenance. I was surrounded by a huge number of people in the school, hospital, and in public, in the city of New Orleans. This was an "intense" psychological time for me in *regard to body image*, caused in part by the unexpected response by people to my new appearance.

I was a very family oriented person, active as an evangelical Christian, and strongly rooted in a good marriage. After overcoming early problems in our marriage we had enjoyed a wonderful family life for about ten years. Al lived another five years after my weight loss. I had no desire to look at another man. Infidelity is one problem that Al and I never had and I am grateful for that. However, I started wearing cute, young clothes, because suddenly I could! I changed my hairstyle. I got mono-vision contact lenses so that I would not have to use reading glasses. My mom said, "Pam has re-invented herself," so great was the outward change in my appearance. My husband just loved it!

Al and I were walking hand in hand one day at a shopping center. One of his old friends from work saw him. She called the house later and asked who he was with at the shopping center. She thought he had gotten himself a girlfriend! Well, Al loved that!

When I told Al that I was very, very uncomfortable in New Orleans with a very visible "knee jerk" reaction from men at times, he just thought it was great. It tickled him because he totally trusted me and he was so proud of the self-confidence I was building. When he married me I was at a slender stage and he loved my little shape.

A good female friend was being very unfriendly and mean to me. She was a beautiful, slender friend. When I began to cry about these new and perplexing problems, Al knew it was serious. He told me to go to a counselor at the medical school and see if she could help me get through this. I had become self-conscious and too focused on myself and my appearance. It was not a comfortable new feeling to deal with and I wasn't sure what to do with it. I did not mean to offend my best friend. However, it became apparent that this good friend needed an obese girlfriend, not another one to compete with. My heart was torn out.

**This is what my counselor said and it is worth sharing to help others who may face the same problem: "Pam, give yourself time…take yourself off the hook about having to get used to this right now. Give yourself <u>time</u> to adjust."**

That advice really helped me, and I did just that. I needed **time** to get used to the new me, the image I suddenly saw in the mirror, and the new image the public had of me. I still carried around the old image, and it would take time to adjust; there was simply no quick fix. I had to give up being in a hurry to get use to this.

Also, **she said:** "Pam, if you live long enough, you will have this body image *challenge again.*" I have had a number of elderly people come into my therapy office for counseling who are dealing with this for the very first time in their lives. For years, they were reasonably attractive and very productive people in many areas of their lives. Suddenly, they have lost some of their identity by no longer working in their careers and physical changes brought on by the aging process. Basically, they don't look on the outside like they feel on the inside. They are greatly troubled by the "general response" in society to their appearance. They need some help dealing with the very unfair reality that they are still the same exact people they once were.

The different response they receive from all people in life is "very tangible," very noticeable.. They are not self-focused people, but are observant enough to see this major change in response to their appearance.

And so, *"Pam, if you live long enough, you will deal with a whole new body image problem once again in your life."* UPDATE! 2020 *The counselor was right. I am dealing with this now at age 69.*

Both of my counselor's points made a huge impact on me. I only went to her once. With Al's help, and praying to get over this, I gave myself time, and in about three years I felt normal, as if I had always been this way. The response I got from men and women no longer bothered me. After you lose a lot of weight and get in shape, some women may feel that you are now in their "competitive" circle; those are the ones that really confused me.

A **very** helpful tool that God put in my mind over this struggling body image was my mother. She had **always** had a wonderful figure, great legs and a very cute face. She knew nothing different! When the family went to the beach, she is the one who got "wolf whistles," not the three girls! She never seemed to notice it, perhaps because this response was what she *had been used to all her life.*

I decided to try and **pretend** that I was "Mom," and that I had felt good about the way I looked **all** my life. Thinking of her helped me a lot, and finally I got into the mindset of just enjoying better health, mobility, and not being so *self-conscious and self-absorbed as Mother had **never** been.* It took **time** to get there, but I finally became used to and comfortable with the new body image.

**It is important to attain a balanced and true reality of your body image, without too much self-focus.**

**But, <u>give yourself time</u>.**

# CHAPTER TWO

## *THE TRUTH WILL SET YOU FREE BUT FIRST IT WILL MAKE YOU MISERABLE!*

These are many of my personal psychological and spiritual discoveries, and more divine interventions. Some thoughts run into other thoughts ….. but I hope I can define for you the very kind and patient leadership of the Holy Spirit, who leads into all truth, if we just listen! *We can regain the truth that we lost earlier in life, and Truth does exist in this area!* I hope that some of my many thoughts are **useful** to your own faith journey in weight loss and **lifetime** weight maintenance.

*God will never reveal more truth about Himself till you obey what you already know.*[4]

**Oswald Chambers**

### *Section One: God's "permissive will" and God's "perfect will."*

**In the hospital room on the night of the surgery in 1995 I really felt that I would die on the operating table. Actually, I felt that I deserved to die, but I knew my children needed me. I thought back to 1980 and my gastric-stapling surgery, also touted for years as a "foolproof" solution to obesity.** It was more like being run over by a car. The recovery was nothing less than horrible. I was opened up from my sternum to my pelvis… no laser surgery existed at that time and the mortality rate was substantial. This surgery would prove as bad or worse, but I felt that God did not want me to live and

---

[4] Quote from Oswald Chambers, from book "My Utmost for His Highest."

act like a seventy-five-year-old woman when I was still young (forty-five) and should have many active and productive years before me.

In my life, during times of intense prayer, many times God has led me to turn open a page in the Bible which has a verse on it that I need very much just at **that time**. God permits this to happen when I am afraid, confused, or doubting. In the hospital room that night, my

Bible just fell open to a verse in Psalms, a verse I had never seen or heard before. Before my Bible fell open to this verse, I had decided that I would pack my bags and leave the hospital. It was not worth the risk. This is what I saw the instant I looked into my bible.

> *I will not die, but live, and proclaim what the Lord has done. The Lord has chastened me severely, but He has not given me over to death.*
> **(Psalm 118: 17-18)**

I cried as I felt the Holy Spirit embracing and comforting me. The Holy Spirit is always our comforter indeed; no matter how far away we are from God's **perfect will in** an area of our lives. I embraced the verse to which my Bible had fallen open, although moments before I had been nearly incapacitated with fear. **It gave me the unsurpassable peace that God would not let me die from the surgery, yet the rest of the verse confused me. I wondered at that time how God might plan to use me because I was cheating by having a "foolproof" obesity surgery where I would not have to work on my problems** (that is what I was told). How would this be a testimony? What did this mean?

As a Christian, I did not feel this surgery route was anything to brag about or encourage others to do. It was unacceptable socially at that time. I was asking for God's mercy and help as He provided this miracle, which was **only in His kind, permissive, will, certainly not in his perfect will of how He made us.**

Remember, at that time in 1995, this surgery was not presented as a "tool." It was presented over and over as a total and permanent miracle-cure to obesity, which I now accept as an innocent overconfidence by the surgeons. **I embraced that this as foolproof just like the promotions indicated. This was my last hope because** I had failed so many times. My husband had the same story.

Back to that very frightening night in 1995 before this major, risky surgery. At that time, in my emotional state, I had to believe without a doubt that I was receiving a lasting miracle from God, and that I would **not** have to work at it. God understood this weakness that I had and how embedded and helpless I was.

**God, in His wonderful, merciful "permissive will" allowed me to believe in that hospital room that all I had to do was to follow the instructions for at least four months in order for the surgery to heal.** Then, for the rest of my life it would be "easy sailing" and I would never be on the dieting roller-coaster again. "Physician assisted starvation" forever!

YAY! Well, I have not been on the roller coaster again, but it was not easy and it was not starvation, thank goodness! I am as healthy as anyone could be with good food, plenty of it in small portions thanks to surgery, and consistent exercise in moderation. I changed my BRAIN! **Eventually, I forgot HOW to be food addicted!**

### *Section Two: Moving on*

No matter how deeply-rooted this problem may be in one's childhood, I firmly believe we can all "move on" beyond the childhood hurts. **My childhood is detailed in Chapter Nine.** We do not have to remain victimized by our deep-seated earlier traumas. We **can truly change our way of thinking** and behaving.

> *"Weight maintenance begins with the mind, not with a diet, and certainly not with a scalpel on the operating table."*[5]
>
> **Tracy Asmussen, my sister**

I definitely feel that a relationship with Christ makes all the difference in order to have the strength to apply these points. A relationship with Christ is not synonymous with regular church attendance or good behavior. It implies a total trust in Jesus Christ and a reliance on the mercy and grace of God in our private lives. Although my husband and I had a deep relationship with Christ over many years, we *still* had this ongoing problem with obesity. Why? Quite simply as Christians still growing in our faith we did not "listen" to

---

[5] Original quote from Tracy Asmussen in Germany. Sociologist, Teacher, my sister.

God's leadership. We refused to have *patience* and used rapid weight loss diets **159 times. They worked every time!**

> *Simply wait upon God. So doing, we shall be directed, supplied, protected, corrected, and rewarded!*[6]
> 
> **Vance Hayner**

Al loved the quote:

*"Vanity is a short-term motivator, while health is the long-term motivator".*

Since Al was loved by everyone who ever knew him, he was not so concerned about how he looked. His greatest worry was not being there for his children, and he deeply regretted not getting his obesity under control sooner. His prayers were answered in that he got to "polish off" his two young adults before he died. My son and my daughter are **real standouts** in character, career, marriage and do not have food addiction! I owe that to Al's last days!

Although we were very ashamed of our past failures and the impending surgery, we felt that God was leading us. God was with us, knowing us completely and knowing what really needed to be done to permanently help us. **God already knew that He would take me to the total truth just one step at a time.** I only knew at that time what "I had" ….. I did not know what "God had." I didn't know it, but the Holy Spirit would

---

[6] Vance Haynor's Devotions

not only be my comforter during this time, but my "counselor" as well. He would lead me and guide me to a lasting solution (which clearly would **not** be the surgery **alone,** though I did not **suspect** this at the time.)

God, through the very hard work that *He required me to do*, transformed the surgery into a lasting tool for me. I was only in God's "permissive will" for the surgery, which often does not lead to a lifetime of lasting, peaceful results. However, God teaches us and develops us during times of His *permissive will*. He knows us from the inside out.

God never lets go of us while trying to lead us into his perfect will and perfect principles, which indeed produce lasting peace and greater joy in our daily lives. The biblical principles regarding health, fitness, money, relationships, and food will <u>not</u> change. <u>We</u> must change in order to live by these principles and to enjoy the harvest of blessings these disciplines bring to our lives!

**Romans 12:1** *"Present your bodies a living sacrifice, holy and acceptable to God."*

**First Corinthians 6:12** *"Everything is permissible to us, but not everything is beneficial. Therefore I will not be enslaved to anything."*

God did not *design our bodies to have an "issue"* with nutrition or exercise. We use to burn off the calories by planting and harvesting our food! This problem is rooted in an industrialized society with cars, phones, desk jobs and convenient foods and drive through restaurants in our hurried lives!

God knew that I had no patience and *He understood how this came about*. I feel that many of us are *victimized by our society*, which contributes to a sedentary lifestyle. We used to burn our calories by regular daily work before so many amenities were available. **I developed a food disorder as an innocent child, when doctors told my mom that certain foods were forbidden for me in order to keep my weight down. This deprivation in childhood worked against me. This was nailed into my psychological development by adulthood.** However, in adulthood, I was certainly the one who had to be responsible to overcome these problems.

God knew that only His principals would set me free forever. He loved me so much that He never gave up trying to reach me. He saw me as an innocent child developing poorly in these areas. He had never condemned me because he knew that wounded and perplexed child was still in me, but He kept convicting me. He allowed His "permissive will" to **start** me in the right direction with this surgery, and led me eventually to his perfect will in this area of life. **In my opinion His perfect will is so simple and so easy and it is one paragraph as follows:**

*Eat a wide variety of foods and especially the low calorie veggies with high fiber, in volume. This will keep you full and in your calorie boundaries. Treat yourself to richer foods (proteins and fats) in smaller percentages. Walk a lot. Use your muscles so you don't lose them! So simple!*

*Did that paragraph require a manual or a book of some type? No! We have lost sight of the wonderful simplicity of how we are made and we let the dieting industry make money off of us because our enemy has stolen our minds on this!*

In my humble lay person's opinion, God's perfect will, with regards to physical health, can be "deduced" from scriptures in the Bible and general history and theological research. This is walking on a regular basis and eating a wide variety of healthy foods. Jesus probably ate wild meats which are lean (a lot of fish, no doubt) breads, veggies, some simple carbs such as fruit, and even bread with honey. And, Jesus walked!

Earlier in the Bible, the children of Israel, as they walked in the desert, were rained down plentiful amounts of "manna." This manna, in Christian research, is said to be whole grain bread, even with a little honey in it! It gave the people the energy they needed to walk, and walk some more. (Complex carbs are our most efficient source of fuel, stored as glycogen in the liver. Glycogen is our most efficient fuel source for aerobic activity, which includes walking.) At night, a much *lesser amount* of protein was rained on them —wild birds, rich in protein and lean in fat.

With a lot of liberty, I would *gleefully* call this "Choosemyplate" as scientists study it today! ChoosemyPlate.gov is over half complex carbs, and the other half is divided between fat and protein. Fat is designed by God to transport hormones and for temperature regulation. Protein is designed by God to build bones, muscle, and hair. This food supply gave them all they needed for their bodies. You can be sure there was no obesity in this group, even though their diets consisted of over 50% carbs, including a simple carb, honey.

Counting carbs is a diet and if you are doing it, you are still trapped in the dieting mentality. If you are convinced that carbs is the cause of your weight problem, and then you have simply not been eating a balance of foods, and probably not with portion/ calorie control. This lack of control creates too many calories, whether they come from carbs or elsewhere. When you go over the edge and as a result **make carbs an outright devil**, you are setting yourself up for failure again and again. **God** made complex carbs, and even a small amount of simple carbs, to be our **greatest source of energy.** If Jesus ate bread; so can you! (Of course, the bread then was not over processed. Make good bread choices and don't eat too much of it.) Too many calories and not enough exercise make us fat, plain and simple (See Chapter six experts). In my opinion a lot of the re-gain in surgery patients are as a result of "the dietary restrictions from the bariatric clinics." There will be restrictions, but pray about the lifetime balance! I have maintained without a legalistic dieting mentality. The first several months of course after surgery, all the restrictions are extremely important in order to recover from the surgery.

***1 Samuel 30:1-6*** *David had reached the point in life where some people think of taking their own lives. He was so far down the ladder of despair that he'd reached the bottom rung. The last stop. The place where you either jump off into oblivion or you cry out to God for His forgiveness. For rescue. The wonderful thing is that we do have that choice, because God never gives up on His children...Dark days call for right thinking and vertical focus. That's what David learns at this moment in his life. He finds that the test isn't designed to throw him on his back and suck him under; it's designed to bring him to his knees so he will look up."*[7]

### Section Three: Let's move forward psychologically and spiritually.

Author Mary Demuth says in one of her devotions:

*We seek comfort in our chains because we have grown so accustomed to them. Perhaps the past was so painful that it "defined us"...Even so, new adventures with Jesus await us. I, for one, am learning to let go of who I was, embracing all God is doing today. So onward and upward we climb and climb and climb... Our faces turn forward with holy anticipation of the rivers of God's presence, spilling into our lives. Will we not perceive it?*[8]

---

[7] Charles Swindolls Internet Devotions

[8] Charles Swindolls Internet Devotions

For those of us who have addictive traits, we may never know exactly how this developed. Others who do not suffer with addictive tendencies just don't understand what it is like to live in our skin. However, I have come to believe that we don't need to delve too deeply (and stagnate there) into the psychological roots of our obsessive and addictive behavior. An encouraging scripture in this regard is: *Philippians 3:13 "Forgetting what is behind, and straining toward the goals which are ahead."*

The negative roots are only a section of our brain. With the right approach, we can "re-program" these sections of our brain. We first need to identify the "practical trigger roots" which manifest this problem.. We can change, even though change is hard. We can conquer the change if we seek the Lord. He will provide the means and His supernatural strength if we are willing to walk out the process with **patience.**

***Romans 8:37-39*** *No, in all these things we are more than conquerors through Him who loved us. For I am convinced that neither death nor life, neither angels nor demons, neither the present nor the future, nor any powers, neither height nor depth, nor anything else in all creation, will be able to separate us from the love of God that is in Christ Jesus our Lord. (Nor any deception by diets!)*

### Section Four: Our hearts have to change first.

A former pastor gave a series of sermons for Christians who want to have more power in all areas of their lives. A quote which resounded with me was: "Our hearts have to change first, and then we have to work on our minds."9 Our minds can, in some respects, be likened to the most powerful computer in the world. They are "programmed" early on and though we may try to purge our learned negative thinking, such thoughts may still pop up unexpectedly on the monitor when you least expect them! However, just as we can change real computer memory and the software, we can change our minds and we can change them perfectly. It just takes time, patience, and the right series of procedures. **I am the worst-case scenario that I know and I have worked with many obese clients over the years. Yet, my mind and thinking changed totally and completely.** So can yours! God does not "zap" us and fix all of our problems with magic.

> *He guides and teaches us; and mercifully. He only lets us see a few areas at a time which need attention so that we are not discouraged and overwhelmed by the task at hand.*
> **Tracy Asmussen**

Joyce Meyer is a Christian author who has written books that would help anyone. She appears on TV each day on her worldwide program "Enjoying Everyday Life." She says "Where the mind goes, the man follows." Once, I heard her say, "Spend time on replacing those empty or bad places in your mind with good things." God did not "zap her" in order to remove all terrible areas of damage in her own life (she was sexually abused for years by her father.) She had to do the hard work and God gave her the strength and patience to do so.

---

[9] Bible Church in Mandeville, LA

I spent a **lot of time on good, new activities that eventually replaced the negatives.** I had to work hard on building up the good, new things in order to "crowd out" the bad habits. **And so, I began to fill up that space in my mind with good stuff until there was no more room for the bad thoughts to move back in. In other words, I focused on making positive changes, instead of focusing so much on the negatives still present.** The enslaving, serious food and exercise problems have never appeared on my screen again even though 24 years have passed with many, many challenges in life, and even though I am "old" now. God in his infinite wisdom knows that you will flounder many times. But He will help you with continuing to climb up that hill and go on to ever new levels, making sure you are on solid ground first with the recent changes.

*The intensity of this struggle that feels powerless can be over. The new habits and forgetting how to do the old ones can become automatic.*

### You can "forget how" to be enslaved to the old habits.

Once God has helped you not only to learn and apply skill powers, but that you are totally enjoying the freedom that this brings, you will feel as if there is just not an "issue" over this problem. God never made this to be an issue. We are victims of this society which gives us no reason to move and little reason to eat well. You will laugh and be amazed it was ever an issue! Your many good habits, (just as in housework, work ethics, or finances), will bring joy and stability.

## Section Five: What's controlling your mind?

I eventually came to the realization that issues with food controlled my mind and in a way actually enslaved me. It robbed me of energy when I needed it. Food was a consolation for stress, fatigue, and boredom. Yet I eventually had to admit that I still had stress and fatigue even after I used food to console myself. It only gave me a few instants of relief, and then it stole my life more and more thoroughly as time went on. I learned to say to me as a kind of mantra, "This momentary use of food will not relieve my stress."

I began to take better care of practical things in life so that there would be less stress and fatigue in my daily life. I began to simplify my life as much as I could. **I accepted that I did not have to be president of everything and on every committee. I became responsible to remove as much stress in my life as possible, instead of using it as an excuse for bad habits.**

### HALT METHOD

*One effective defense against temptation is to know **when** we are weak. Satan often strikes after waiting for us to reach our physical and emotional limits... Wise believers avoid becoming too hungry, angry, lonely, or tired (HALT). Letting oneself reach such extremes opens the door for Satan's short-term solutions, like an unwise business deal or an unsuitable marriage partner.*[10]

Dr. Charles Stanley – In Touch

---

[10] In Touch Magazine July 2007

I remember the HALT warning often and have taken it to heart. Elaborations in regard to the "HALT" acronym are from me and not from Charles Stanley, but his HALT acronym has been a significant support for me over the years. (HALT- hungry, angry, lonely, tired)

At all costs, I practice the avoidance of unnecessary stress because I identified this is a **major trigger for me.** I had to **rearrange my life** in order to achieve a reduction in stress through simplification of my lifestyle. At times, I have to remind myself to repeat the simplification process when I notice a sudden increase in daily stress.

While losing the weight, though I needed the money, I quit my job for six months; and I discontinued ministries and volunteer work. I had to face the fact that I had never been able to succeed in an exercise program because I was too busy and stressed out to follow one consistently. I explained to everyone that I needed to put my body and health as a first priority for at least the next year, and then I would return to activities as God led me. I truly believed that my drastic decision was the best way I could serve God and delete this compulsive behavior from my life. (Later, I trusted God to find me the best and highest paying job I had ever had in my life, which I had the **new found confidence to apply for because of some weight loss!**)

About two years after I had *maintained* my weight loss for a solid year, I returned to one ministry at church. I also worked on motivational speaking to the public. However, I still keep my life simple, not overworked or overstressed. Most importantly, and it is usually women who have to pay heed to this, I have learned to say "No!" I feel that as I go through this world I am a more effective Christian when I am not stressed out, even if I am not on every committee in the church. I focus on my true callings by God, and am no longer a "jack of all trades" being unable to <u>say no</u> to areas of community or church service which are outside of my own personal stress level. Therefore, I stay much more effective to the "everyday" opportunity to show God's love. Those are opportunities that I use to ignore as I was too busy to show love as I go!

We can all become victims or a hurried life style without realizing it. If you have no time to take care of your body by way of a regular, consistent exercise program; if you have no time to stop and shop and make reasonable food choices which are best for your health, then more than likely something in your life needs to be dropped. I have heard and seen hundreds of examples of this from clients. As I trained clients, I could see a big problem is the "hurried lifestyle." You can improve on this, no matter what your present situation. Some stages of life are naturally more stressful, but you can even improve on those. Whatever you do, don't use these times of stress as an excuse for neglecting your health, as my husband and I did.

Whatever you do, <u>don't beat yourself up</u> when you have a day or a week when you absolutely had no control over a horrible stressful time, with no time to take care of yourself and perhaps you used food. If you have a bariatric pouch, it is much easier to recover! Be grateful for that! Just say to yourself, "I got a lot done, I had my priorities right before

God's eyes, and **'starting over' tomorrow or this week on my exercise and food program is 'just awesome.'"**

Joyce Meyer teaches about "battle position." My "battle position" in overcoming these problems was in working on other areas of my life either first during that "time out" that the new surgery gives. Be sure you are in "battle position" and take advantage of this time out.

I highly recommend the book, *100 Ways to Simplify Your Life*, by Joyce Meyer.

### Section Six: The four P's: Prayer, Preparation, Planning, and Patience

I used these four concepts daily to change my life. I still use them. Through this continual, verbal prayer and listening to God, I began to believe that life could be simpler, on many levels, and entail less stress. In 1996, I began to believe that God wanted simplification for me, and He would provide the opportunities if I would take them. To achieve this simplification required a lot of initial preparation and planning on my part; now, it only requires maintenance. The list of suggestions on how to go about this is too long to print here. I am sure there are many books available with endless examples for simplifying one's life.

We will always have some stress; it comes with the job of living; but if we take time to rethink how we live and what our personal stressors are, **we can plan** *much of the stress out of our lives and build stress-relievers in. I became very conscious* *of this and did the hard work to prevent as much of it as possible.*

### Section Seven: SUPERNATURAL OPPOSITION must be overcome with SUPERNATURAL MEANS

Prayer should be continual and, believe me, **God is listening.** He is also **trying to make us listen to Him.**

> *For the weapons of our warfare are not worldly, but are mighty through God to the pulling down of <u>strongholds</u> in our lives. Casting out imaginations and bringing into captivity <u>every thought into the</u> <u>obedience</u> of Christ.*
>
> **2 Corinthians 10:4-5 NKJV**

We have all heard, "we reap what we sow." God continues to love us and reach out to us, but consequences must be paid because these principals are laid out in the Bible, and they are not going to change.

*With God, we are free to choose what we surrender to, but we are not free from the consequences of the choice.*

*Remember, if we don't give up, we make progress (progress, not perfection).*

*Our "building blocks" become so strong that the struggle becomes easier.*

## HURRICANE KATRINA

- **Transfer addictions for the addictive personality. BEWARE!!**

- **How I found my children after the storm.**

After Hurricane Katrina I was gripped with brand new obsessive / addictive oral behavior. This new struggle helped me recall the agonizing details of how hard I had worked to change my mindset and behavior in the past. Katrina allowed me to remember that real change takes a long time and is the result of hard work; rarely the result of a single "zap" from God.

**The new Addiction**: Around a year before the hurricane, during the summer of 2004, I had started puffing on an apple-flavored cigar about three times a week after dinner while sitting on the porch with my new condo neighbors. I hardly inhaled and it was a nice kickback with neighbors. I did this discreetly as to not be a "stumbling block" to anyone who did not approve of this fairly benign habit. There was nothing about this after dinner cigar, a *few* times weekly, that I felt affected my life, my health, or my witness, as long as it was just with my neighbors. Many people are able to puff on a cigar and not become enslaved to it. I never would have touched a cigarette because I did not like the taste of it, thank God. These cigars were flavored, almost like an after dinner small dessert. It eased the disappointment and severe loneliness I was feeling over a potential second-marriage opportunity that had failed. I had sworn off dating and just stayed at home evenings after dinner. It eased the loneliness after supper that I felt without Al and the children being the focus of my daily life.

After Katrina, I consoled myself even more with the apple-flavored cigars, and they eventually became another addiction; it was no longer just a private kickback. I certainly *understand* almost any oral addiction now, after opening myself up to this particular one. It can safely be said that "moderation" became a thing of the past for many Hurricane Katrina victims, including Christians. The overwhelming stress and grief that many suffered at that time simply drove a lot of people over the edge. A side, but related point: some people who lose a lot of weight are immediately faced with brand new obsessive/ addictive behavior right after their initial weight loss. We have an obsessive/addictive personality trait down inside of us and it simply transfers to another habit. This new behavior of cigars only hit me a *full nine years after the surgery.* Therefore, I would not say it was the "typical transfer addiction" since it occurred as long after the weight loss as it did. (Hurricane Katrina was not typical as well!) However, I believe it was a "transfer addiction." I am now aware of my personality and that despite my powerful faith in Christ, **I must stay away from any arena that even remotely seduces me and could cause enslaving oral habits.**

Two years after the storm, I had an unusually large number of clients who were obese for the very first time. Many of them were wonderful Christian people who knew their Bibles well and praised God for all their answered prayers. But, like me, they had a propensity to sedate themselves with something oral. People who do not have this tendency certainly do not understand.

Many people used food to get through the long, long aftermath of Hurricane Katrina. Some of them had never even been on a diet! They were very miserable, to say the least, with this new problem. I saw them as clients after the Hurricane.

For me, before this new habit of the cigars became truly enslaving, it eased the *after-supper, nighttime* loneliness for a real partner, which I had enjoyed for thirty years, the majority of my adult lifetime. No longer being a wife and active mother was still a new challenge to me.

I was more alone and miserable once I moved to my FEMA apartment in another state (Oregon.) People evacuated to various places to live between four months and a couple of years, with the help of FEMA, Red Cross, and others. My daughter Tiffany and her husband Brad were distraught at not even being allowed to go home to New Orleans (I live thirty-five miles north of them) and I was filled with worry over their situation. We each lost a lot materially and the **future was totally uncertain with regards to lost jobs, housing, and virtually, everything we take for granted in life, although we suffered less than many others and were daily thankful for what we had not lost. Because of the mass destruction and millions of** claims, it took two months to even see an insurance adjustor and another year before all our insurance money came in. It took two years to finish every last repair on my waterfront condo, situated on a bayou but a whole mile from the lake. The millions of claims and shortages on contractors made this disaster very different from any other. *I did not return to overeating to relieve this stress, but had a cigar in my hand everywhere! My new addiction... hopeless, powerless to overcome it.*

**How I found my precious daughter, Tiffany and her precious husband, Brad after the storm.**

For three days following the hurricane's major strike on New Orleans and surrounding areas, I could not locate my daughter and her husband who lived in New Orleans, and who as it turned out were stranded at her in-law's **two story** house in Slidell, Louisiana, nine feet of water on the first floor.... a lake! There was no way to communicate. Tiff and Brad were responsible for his elderly parents in a storm. Tiff and Brad had successfully evacuated New Orleans, where they lived and worked, before the storm and they live there even now. No phones were working at the time, and I was desperate for news of them. After waiting three days for a rescue that never came, and giving out of drinking water, they finally swam out on their own strength once the water had receded to four feet because her elderly father in-law required medical attention. I did everything I could to get into Slidell and see if I could find her, although most streets were blocked and no one was allowed in due to downed trees, power lines, and flood waters. I went to shelters for the homeless and could not believe I did not see their sweet faces! I was determined not to let that stop me, and once again drove two hours west of us to get gasoline, as there was no gas anywhere near me. In the gasoline line, at least a *mile long* extending into the highway, I heard an excited voice a distance away, shouting,

"Mama H!" It was my son-in-law's voice! Suddenly I heard my daughter screaming, "Let me out!" Her door was locked and she couldn't figure out how to unlock it, being in a borrowed van. Tiffany ran down the interstate and the two of us stood there hugging with relief for the longest time. Eventually, she had to tell me to let go of her! She and Brad had hitchhiked out of Slidell, Louisiana and ended up in the same long gas line as myself in another town! There had been no way to communicate... because cell phone towers were damaged. There were others who were not so fortunate, and being aware of that, we could only thank God we had been spared the loss of life in our family. They returned that night and rescued Brad's parents themselves as there were no other rescuers yet in their area. I told Tiffany, "Please let the rescuers get Brad's parents."

She looked at me with glassed over eyes, and said, "There are no rescuers, Mom." The man who had given them a lift on the highway had just dug out of his **one story** house through the roof. Luckily his van was parked at the hospital where his wife was a nurse. The friend had watched his beloved dogs drown one at a time, because they could no longer tread water. He would not talk about the dogs. Slidell, Louisiana did not get much attention. The attention was on New Orleans for a long time. Tiff, Brad, and the man who gave them a ride were in neighborhoods that were *safe*. They did not **even require flood insurance. Their houses were miles away from the Lake, not anywhere near "lakefront property."**

*We were grateful that our lives were saved, but the long-term emotional distress and the long-term financial uncertainty over lost income and living arrangements was not to be so easily ignored.*

Certainly, many people took up new and often negative habits just to survive daily and combat the extreme stress we were all under. Many people who had never before taken blood pressure medication, or had never experienced clinical depression, were now having these problems among many others. An increased suicide rate was also reported beginning about a year after the storm.

Thankfully, I did not use food to face this unusual level of stress which is quite rare, something I had never before encountered, and hope never again to endure. If it was a final test to see how far I had come in my battle against using food for emotional relief, then I passed with flying colors.

But I did nevertheless end up becoming addicted to the cigars, something I still *cannot believe I succumbed* to. However, once I became fully aware of my addiction, I decided to get this new habit out of my life. It took two years to rid myself of this as a habitual enslavement, and I will never forget how easily I was "fooled" to fall into the trap of hopeless addiction again!

No matter how much we love the Lord and follow Him, I suggest to all Christians **not to overestimate your spiritual strength** as we all live in "jars of clay;" (2 Corinthians 4:7) because then you can fall into something that diminishes your witness and your energy to serve Him. We are ALL one thought away from temptation in this earthly environment we are in. Beware!

So, I had hard work to do once again in simplifying my life, praying, obeying, and getting back to God as *number one*. I had to be very patient in overcoming this new problem. I called upon the personal skills I had developed when learning new attitudes and habits in the areas of food and exercise, which is why I say I could not have defined the message in this chapter in this much detail without going through the misery of Katrina;

I had simply *forgotten how hard it was to overcome an enslaving emotional and stress related habit. It is much better to stay away from those things initially.*

The following is from Dr. Charles Stanley "In Touch" magazine.

This article illustrates how I often felt with addictions:

*"A Christian sometimes becomes convinced that God's forgiveness has limits. Satan whispers in our ear continually that the Lord had to be weary of this constant sin/admission cycle. As always, the Enemy lies. Jesus' sacrifice on the cross paid our past, present and future sin-debt. He forgives sin as often as necessary if we ask. He shows us where we have grown wrong and how we can correct our actions to return to the path of righteousness. God desires that each of us grow in righteousness and reflect the nature of his son Jesus Christ. He understands that maturing our faith is a lifelong process. Sometimes we will make mistakes and fall into sinful patterns from which we must be restored. Our Father is pleased to draw us back into a right relationship because*

*his grace is infinite. No sin will ever be greater – or more frequent – than God's capacity to forgive us and continue to teach us."*

**Charles Stanley**

God is more interested in developing the workman, than developing the actual work." He wants to develop character in us as we go, much more than propel us quickly to reach the final goal of all the weight loss. Character involves patience, humility, and self-control; God wants to develop all these traits in us while we are waiting and working toward final victory.

# CHAPTER THREE

## *METABOLISM AND GENETICS*

The facts presented in this chapter were not "invented" by any medical doctor. They are simply facts pertaining to human physiology that have not been subject to change for thousands, if not millions, of years.

A Basal Metabolic Rate is the number of calories burned at rest in a twenty-four hour period. This includes the calories needed for digestion, sleep, respiration; our basal metabolism affects how fast we can break down and burn the calories we consume.

The good news is we can change a poor BMR slowly by having a formal exercise program. Everybody has the right to know how many calories they should consume daily and how to burn these calories efficiently. The BMR formula is an excellent guide to find your proper caloric intake and also to maintain your desired weight as well as for weight loss or weight gain.

Two ways to affect our BMR are through a properly balanced diet and formal exercising. The amount of lean body mass we have can change through age, sickness, or exercise – lean body mass affects the BMR.

*Table 9-1 Factors that affect Basal Metabolic Rate (Hamilton/Whitney's Textbook, Sixth Edition)*

| FACTOR | EFFECT ON BMR |
|---|---|
| Age | In youth, the BMR is higher; age brings less lean body mass and slows the BMR. |
| Height | Tall, thin people have higher BMR's. |
| Growth | Children and pregnant women have higher BMR's. |
| Body Composition | The more lean tissue; the higher the BMR. |
| Fever | Fever raises the BMR. |
| Stress | Stress hormones raise the BMR. |
| Environmental temp. | Both heat and cold raise the BMR. |
| Fasting/Starvation | Fasting/Starvation **hormones lower** the BMR. |
| Malnutrition | Malnutrition lowers the BMR. |
| Thyroxin | The thyroid hormone thyroxin is a key regulator; the more Thyroxin produced, the higher the BMR. |

My BMR was affected by height, and further mutilated by fasting/starvation and malnutrition from diets, all induced by diet doctors from childhood. This included using amphetamines prescribed by doctors for years in childhood. I was on the playground on "speed" and did not eat much food or good nutrition at all in order to be thin. Many women my age have this same story.

At age thirty I was diagnosed with a very, very low thyroid, resulting from problems with the pituitary gland. They told me the symptoms of "childhood" low thyroid and I had them all from age six years old, including constipation. As a child, I was tested for low thyroid, but they did **not have** the **pituitary test** at that time. So, my entire childhood was with a very low amount of thyroxin being produced by the pituitary gland to send to the thyroid gland. In addition to childhood constipation as a symptom, other symptoms are sluggishness, short stature, and depression. Therefore, it was not "my entire fault" that weight was a struggle for me. I had "professional" help with the starvation medication and a "genetic disposition" from the very low thyroid and height listed in the table! I am convinced that this also contributed to the severe psychological problems I had as a child and teenager. Many of you need to stop beating yourselves up and realize that it is not all your fault either. However, it was **all my responsibility** to do something about it and that is possible. I hope that you will accept the challenge also! For many of you, like me, a primary resolution would be to have pride in a good, healthy weight and a cute shape. Many of us with a slower BMR, for whatever reasons, will not be able to acquire "thinness".

I am also qualified on the chart to be affected by **age,** despite my good lifestyle. I will continue to do all I can, but be accepting of my age! I refuse to be obese at an older age, after losing so much time at a younger age!

### *Nutshell Study: Moseby Yearbook January, 1998*

This yearbook is a very respected medical book. This synopsis has not changed 24 years later. You can find this book in medical libraries. You can Google!

# Basal Metabolic Rate (Moseby Yearbook)

Basal metabolic rate accounts for most of a person's calorie use. A person's basal metabolic rate is based on body functions such as respiration, digestion, heartbeat, and brain function. (the age, sex, body weight, and the type of physical activity impact the basal metabolic rate. Basal metabolic **rate increases** with the amount of muscle tissue a person has, and it **reduces** with age (we lose muscle starting about age 30).

Along with the use of calories, the basal metabolic rate is increased during physical activity and also **after** the physical activity. The basal metabolic rate can remain increased to 24 – 48 hours after 40 minutes of moderate type of physical activity. For many people the basal metabolism can **be increased 10% for approximately 48 hours after the activity.**

**Note from Pam:** Aren't those **extra** calories that we burn when we are **sleeping** or watching TV more exciting than the ones on the treadmill? These facts highly motivated me towards frequency years ago in my power walking program.

Nancy Clark is a Registered Dietician, and a nutrition counselor at Boston Area Sports Medicine, Brookline. In her book, *Nancy Clark's Sports Nutrition Guidebook*, she says: *The question arises: What is the cost of starvation? What happens to the body and the mind when food is restricted?*

She goes on to cite a study which proves that starvation diets cause a plethora of problems for the dieter and concludes with this disturbing fact:

*Weight is more than a matter of will power. That is, if you lose weight, your body will fight to return to a genetically normal level. We also learn from the study that dieters who restrict to the point of semi-starvation are likely to regain all the weight they lost – plus more.*[11]

This does not have to happen to any Bariatric patient provided they lose the weight slowly on a diet of higher calories, instead of by semi-starvation methods, and practice a moderate and consistent exercise program. All of them want to lose 100 pounds in 4 months. I am so thankful my prayers were ignored on this. On a scale of a One to a Ten, God gave me a Ten, not a Two, in response to my prayers! The price I paid was a slow weight loss, but during that **waiting** time, God trained me and corrected me and changed my brain into a normal response to food and exercise!

### Dieting and Metabolism

Weight Loss Resources dietician, Juliette Kellow, bsc/RD, explains how dieting can affect metabolism and how you can increase your metabolic rate:

---

[11] April 2008, published by Human Kinetics. Nancy Clark, RD, MS Sports Nutrition Guidebook (reliance on all academic information such as macronutrients and how they work in the body) Updated academic information and certification units for trainers are contained in the large educational website of www.nancyclarkrd.com This is a continual educational source for me as I only use Registered Dieticians for kinesiology facts and nutrition facts. She is my primary resource as a certified trainer and I have heard her speak at various national certification classes for Personal Trainers. She educates many trainers.

*"Severely restricting calories actually prevents our bodies from burning unwanted fat stores effectively – and unfortunately, this means that weight loss slows down...quite simply, your body goes into starvation mode. This mechanism, which is thought to have evolved as a defense against starvation, means the body becomes super-efficient at making the most of the calories it does get from food and drink. The main way it does this is to protect its fat stores and instead use lean tissue or muscle to provide it with some of the calories it needs to keep functioning. This directly leads to loss of muscle, which in turn lowers metabolic rate so that the body needs fewer calories to keep ticking and weight loss slows down. Of course, this is the perfect solution if you're in a famine situation. But, if you're trying to lose weight, it's going to do little to help you shift those unwanted pounds.*

*The metabolic rate, the rate at which the body burns calories – is partly determined by the amount of muscle we have. In general, the more muscle we have, the higher our metabolic rate; the less muscle we have, the lower our metabolic rate. This explains why men, who have a high proportion of muscle, have a faster metabolism than women, and why a 20 year old has a higher metabolism than a 70 year old – again, they have more muscle...research shows that the body loses a proportionately high amount of muscle with a very low calorie intake and this may considerably suppress metabolism by up to 45 percent...it is crucial to protect your metabolic rate."*[12]

## Calorie is a beautiful word!

Some hard facts I learned while working in the medical school which impressed me, and which were never emphasized in all my years of dieting, although they are constants, are as follows:

- The scientific term for calorie is "ENERGY." The calorie is a HEAT UNIT.

- The calories in food represent a form of potential energy for our bodies to produce heat and work. Knowing how many calories (that is, energy units) are in our food can reveal how much food we need to perform the work inside our bodies as well as all our movements (daily work, exercise.) If we eat more energy units than we need for all of our functions, we simply store the units (gain fat or weight.) Conversely, if we eat less energy units than we need, the body will draw on its fat stores (lose fat or weight.)

As I studied this, over and over, the word CALORIE became a good word in my vocabulary. In fact, it became a wonderful word! In the past, it was my enemy and instilled fear in me because I was forever dieting on very low calories and, consequently, regaining my weight on low calories as

---

[12] Information from Juliette Kellow, RD, in her website
www.weightlossresources.co.uk/diet/dietitian.htm

well. How I dreaded the fearsome monster CALORIE! Once I learned how to use energy units by embracing enough of them in my diet and expelling some of them through exercise, Calorie became my friend!

I do not expect to ever become a perfect eater, if such thing exists, but I know my caloric and fat gram values and, therefore, have nothing to fear. I am in control. I eat, cheat, and treat based on staying within my calories values. This has helped me to embrace food as my friend and not my enemy. In order to stay full, I eat enough "good foods" with lots of fiber that contribute to bringing my "treats" back into a good average on a food analysis deemed proper by a Registered Dietician (RD). The following is a basal metabolism formula taken from a medical school textbook. A variety of these are printed in many metabolism and nutrition textbooks. I have always used this one. They all come up with similar number results.

If you are aware that you have a lot of muscle, (muscular build), you should also use a body fat analysis before you determine what your desired weight is for your formula. If you have a muscular figure or physique, you can carry more weight and look trim! You can come up in the overweight category on a body mass index chart, while you may look great in person. Some women have more lean body mass than other women and will weigh more on the scale, and appear to be thinner and more compact. The amount of muscle we have is in some part from genetics. We can all build more muscle fiber, though we may not have "great show," by using resistance training and just plain hard work in life.

If you don't go to the trouble to do a body fat analysis as well, just estimate your ideal weight if you are a muscular person by adding five pounds to the chart if you are a woman. Add fifteen pounds to the chart if you are a man. This idea is strictly an estimate from me based on all the thousands of body fat analysis I have done on clients over the years.

## Body Mass Index (BMI)

Body mass index, or BMI, is a new term to most people. However, it is the measurement of choice for many physicians and researchers studying obesity. BMI uses a mathematical formula that takes into account both a person's height and weight. BMI equals a person's weight in kilograms divided by height in meters squared. (BMI=kg/m2). You can google BMI charts.

I am a 24 BMI, (from 1996 to 2012) which I accept fully as my mentally and physically healthy weight. A 24 BMI is at the top of my chart for just being being inside a healthy weight. If I still had no blood profile problems at a 27 BMI, (true from 2012 starting in mid-60s) I *could accept that also,* but I would grow out of my clothes. Clothes are expensive and I love my clothes!!

## FORMULAS for Basal Metabolism (caloric needs)

These formulas are standard formulas used by Registered Dieticians and can be found in college textbooks. They do vary from book to book, but the following are commonly used.

The BMR formula is as follows: I'll use the example of a 150 pound man who is at his ideal weight.

**Your "desired weight" in kilograms divided by 2.2; 150 pounds divided by 2.2 = 68 kilograms**

**Your kilogram weight x 24; 68 x 24 = 1636 calories**

This means this man can eat 1,636 calories daily in order to maintain his desired weight with no formal exercise program.

Subtract 100 calories for females, who have less muscle, and people over forty years old who have lost muscle through the aging process.

1,636 calories does not seem like much, and it's not, but to maintain his 150 pounds and not exercise he would have to stay in this caloric intake range to maintain his weight. He is only 5'6". The good news is this number can be improved by regular exercise and a proper caloric intake. Excessively low calories over duration can lower the BMR. The body will burn muscle as energy and conserve the small number of calories it is getting.

Lost muscle, through fast weight loss, makes maintaining your weight very difficult. Eventually, with a constant unnecessary struggle, we lose the battle.

## Formulas for your use:

### Energy In, Energy Out (Calories ← Calories →)

Your BMR x .30 For the light exerciser Your BMR x .40 For the moderate exerciser Your BMR x .50 For the heavy exerciser

Using the 150 lb. man as an example, I will explain the above formula. He exercises formally 3 ½ hours per week (moderate exerciser). He would take his BMR, which was 1,636 calories – and multiply it by .40.

1,636 x .40 = 654 calories

He could then add 654 calories to his 1,636 = 2,290 calories

On the moderate exercise program, he could maintain his weight of 150 pounds on about 2,300 calories per day. (His "Total Energy Expenditure" amount)

## Weight Loss using your BMR formula:

How can he lose some extra weight and keep it off? To understand this formula we will use this same man's numbers.

His total energy expenditure = 2,290.

He will subtract 500 calories from this amount = 1,790 calories. Consuming around 1,800 calories while still using his moderate exercise program will result in lost weight.

He will not lose lean body mass using these proper numbers and so his BMR will not go lower as it would on a starvation diet, but it will remain good and might even improve. However, this will not be a fast weight loss.

You would add 500 calories to your Total Energy Expenditure to purposely gain weight. Yes, some of my clients have struggled with being underweight!

## Fat Gram Formula

The United States Department of Agriculture, the American Heart Association, and the American Dietetic

Association, and others recommend 20-30% of our caloric intake come from fat. (They also support the "food pyramid" instead of low carb diets by diet doctors.) This fat gram formula allows you to calculate the number of fat grams you need daily to achieve the dietary guidelines set at 20-30% of your calories. On the back of most food labels you will find dietary guidelines based on a 2,000 calorie diet. To make it easy though, I'll use 2,290 calories as an example, from the previous man's example. His fat gram formulas would be different than the following if we used his low amount of 1,800 while he loses weight.

**The formula is calculated as follows: 2,290 calories x .20% =458 458 divided by 9 = rounded off to 50 grams daily**

This will vary depending on your individual calorie requirement in your previous formula. People with a high lipid profile (high cholesterol or triglycerides) should not have 30% but use the low end of 20%, as we did in the example. Remember, you can consume more than 50 grams of fat in just one fast food combo meal!

### *PROTEIN REQUIREMENTS: (BY REGISTERED DIETICIANS WHO STUDY NUTRITION FOR YEARS)*

*Written by Erin Coleman,* **R.D., L.D.***; Updated December 12, 2018*

Protein is an essential nutrient important for growth and development in children and for muscle growth, **repair and maintenance**. Protein is also a structural component of your skin, organs and glands. Consuming too little protein can lead to loss of muscle mass, stunted growth, **fatigue** and changes in your skin and hair.

Your individualized protein requirements are based on your age, gender and activity level.

## Children

Children need protein on a daily basis to grow and develop at a healthy pace. According to the Institute of Medicine:

- babies 0 to 6 months of age need 9.1 grams of protein
- infants ages 7 to 12 months need 11 grams of protein
- children ages 1 to 3 need 13 grams of protein
- kids ages 4 to 8 need 19 grams of protein
- boys and girls ages 9 to 13 need 34 grams of protein
- girls ages 14 to 18 need 46 grams of protein
- boys ages 14 to 18 need 52 grams of protein

## Women, Pregnancy and Breast-feeding

The Institute of **Medicine** recommends all adult women consume at least 46 grams of protein every day. During pregnancy and breast-feeding, a woman's protein requirements significantly increase to 71 grams of protein per day. These are minimum protein requirements, estimated to meet the needs of the majority of women. However, actual protein requirements may be higher, depending on a woman's individualized needs and activity level.

## Men

The recommended dietary allowance for protein for men is 56 grams per day, or 0.8 grams per kilogram of body weight. This equals about 0.36 grams of protein per pound of body weight. Based on the protein RDA, a 170-pound man needs at least 61 grams of protein each day. Active men likely require more protein than this minimum requirement.

## Older Adults

Loss of muscle mass is associated with aging, and is especially prevalent in the senior population. The RDA for older adults is 0.8 grams per kilogram, or about 0.36 grams of protein per pound of body weight per day. However, a review published in a 2015 edition of **Nutrients** reported that older people who consume more protein than the RDA can improve their strength, muscle mass, and bone health and immune status. The review concluded that optimal protein intake for seniors is 1.0 to 1.3 grams per kilogram, or about 0.4 to 0.5 grams of protein per pound of body weight each day.

## Athletes

Athletes require more protein than non-athletes, and the amount of protein needed is based on size and activity level. The Academy of Nutrition and Dietetics reports that endurance athletes need about 0.6 to 0.9 grams of protein per pound, and strength-trained athletes trying to build muscle mass need 0.6 to 0.8 grams of protein per pound of body weight each day.

People need all this information to maintain a healthy heart. They need to do the calculations in the formulas in this chapter. They need to keep simple records on this and discover where they are (my resource page at the end of this book gives webs that will help you!) Since a fat gram has 9 calories per gram, instead of the 4 calories per gram in protein or carbs, just watching fat intake can result in weight loss also. However, remember that fat intake is important and you need no less than 15% for transportation of nutrients, some hormones, etc., as discussed earlier.

### *Genetic Make-up*

A lot of the following phrases and words are studies from my Apex Fitness Professional Manual and this is what makes an Apex Personal Training Club really good. The manual is full of very academic points and teaches a certified trainer a real science, which results in a better program for the client. Some of this is my own interpretation of this academic manual with a paraphrase. The words in italics are verbatim quotes.

Our trillion dollar a year dieting industry is mostly driven by doctors who are blessed with good genetics! When you study the metabolism chart, you can see what really good genetics are: tall and thin, no thyroxin problems, preferably male, etc. Like you, I had none of those benefits to support me physically or mentally in order to create a positive cycle of normal behavior toward food and exercise.

*People who have never had serious roots of abnormal attachment to food and who have always loved the discipline of exercise have been telling us for decades how to think and act about food!* (Apex)

We trust them because they are usually doctors, yet they get only three months of nutrition studies in medical school! This was true when I worked at the medial school with residents and the doctor I worked for told me this is all that was required, unless they were specializing in his field. Nutrition, metabolism, and how movement affects all of that is not something that every doctor is an expert on.

*In other words, we find a large portion of a genetically gifted group, who may not be specialists in this area, instructing the less endowed on how to achieve physical goals. (Apex)*

Also, some trainers allow their clients to believe they will eventually look like them, simply because they are doing the same exercises the trainer uses. I emphasize that trainers should not mislead their clients into thinking this is possible in every instance.

The weight loss challenge shows on TV may not lead to lifetime truth for many people who are watching the shows. They may not lead to lifetime success for many of those on the shows. Grit, willpower, and no cheating are stressed. Exercise has already "progressed" to almost a maximal limit (starting out.) Lifetime moderation, gradual progression in exercise, and permanent changes are not very sensational and do not make a good TV show. This is sensationalism, which for me is nothing more than what fast weight loss doctors have taught for years. You can learn a lot of correct and good values from the shows, but be cautious and remember what I have said! I remember watching the Dr. Phil show one day while three of his alumni from this weight loss challenge show were guests. The contestants lived in a special house while on the show.

The ladies kept asking, "How can I do this forever?.... I am about to face 'real life' once again and I am afraid!"

We want to look like our trainer or Dr. Oz on the Oprah Show! I will never look like most of the other trainers! I will never look like Dr. Oz.

*However, I broke free of the chains of medical obesity by eating just enough calories and exercising just enough. Too little calories or too much exercise can derail the process, slowing down your BMR, or burning you out on exercise. I am realistic about how much I can achieve, based on my own genetics, and I educated myself on the numbers. I did not break free of these chains by the surgery alone. If you have truly reviewed this book in detail, you will understand that and this is important for a pre-op patient, or post-op patient, or anyone who feels that "we have cheated" by using this surgery.* **Fast weight loss that is produced from surgery or any popular Diet Doctor diet, works against many of us physically and emotionally.**

The question I would like to address now is whether it is possible to alter genetic potentials or not? Obviously, it is not possible to modify the genes themselves. An individual's actual genetic predisposition is fixed before birth and cannot be changed.

*However, it is possible to influence whether these genes are allowed to fully express themselves over time. (Apex)*

So, the answer is an optimistic, "Yes!" As already explained in my personal story, at age forty-six I experienced what I felt was a miracle--after years of starving myself and subsequently gaining weight, I discovered that I could eat enough food to satisfy myself and exercise moderately, losing weight slowly and consistently, and eventually I had an improved metabolism. **I was able to eat more than I ever had before and without a painful, burnout exercise program. My weight stopped "jumping up" over the slightest thing**. I stayed the same size all the time. I had never, ever experienced this very "peaceful maintenance" of a healthy weight in my life!

When you have damaged your metabolism, it may take a long time to fully correct it, but it is worth the delay if you are sick and tired of dieting. You must accept a slow weight loss in order to eventually correct your damaged metabolism. In the long run, it is well worth the effort.

I did not lose just 60% of my excess weight as many gastric by-pass patients do, and which is honestly expressed upfront by the surgery clinics themselves. Do you understand that many of these patients have a calorie burn that just comes to a standstill, because they lost 100 or more pounds so fast that their body is trying to "save them" and conserves the calories they are taking in, which are still not many calories?

**Because my *stoma stretched early*,** I was able to have a normal amount of calories and my body *did not go* into "starvation mode." I lost weight until I lost 85% of my excess weight. I stopped there because I had been having just 1,200 calories a day, and I was ready to have more! I was the *fortunate* surgery patient. **The way that we lose affects the way that we maintain.**

"The long-term success of a fast weight loss diet, promoted by most diet doctors, is less than 5%." (Apex Fitness Journal) We don't really need confirmation on that point. All we have to do is just continually observe everyone we know who always gains their weight back after losing a lot fast.

> *Fad diets and fast weight loss diets fail because of the nutritional inadequacies and failure to focus on things people don't want to do – change exercise and eating habits for life. (Apex)*

> *The facts are simple: we are fatter as a society because we consume approximately 300 more calories (energy units) daily than we did two decades ago and we move less because of labor-saving devices.(Apex)*

**In early civilization we hunted for our food, running after it with spears in our hands. Later in civilization, we planted, harvested, and worked for our food. Later, we**

**walked to the store for our food. Now, we drive to the supermarket, or worse, we drive by a little window and pick it up in a bag! The rest of the animal kingdom still burns their food calories in the process of obtaining their food: "Eating and moving, moving and eating." (Apex live seminar)**

I share this with you because many of you are victims of genetics, but you can still overcome your genetic tendencies, just as I did. Many people do not have genes that create a slender build.

While we all appreciate the advantages of living in our modern, industrialized and ultra-convenient society, one of the disadvantages is that we can now quickly and easily put on a good deal of extra weight before we realize what is happening. Those of us with genes that put as at a higher risk for obesity can put on so much extra weight with fast and easy access to high calorie and high fat food that we move into the medically obese category in a matter of a few years.

We do not have to be prisoners or victims of our genes. "Blue Zones" in the world were highlighted in the news this week. They are studies of areas where people live a long time and have different habits than Americans have. The study <u>really proved</u> that we don't have to be victims of our genes. <u>Environment plays a huge role</u>. GOOGLE BLUE ZONES.

*Our genes control appetite, satiety (feeling full and satisfied), basal and exercise metabolism and the point at which excess energy intake is converted into lean tissue or fat. Yet, while there is probably a pre-determined set point range that is heavily influenced by genes, people can and do lose weight and keep it off even if they are in the high-risk category for obesity. Ultimately, we are in control of the numbers, that is, "calories in and out." (Apex)*

I have learned how to do this easily and there are tools for you in this chapter and on my resource page for you to figure out how to do it easily (the way that I had to study it and figure it out years ago.) I have also learned to **accept** some extra pounds on my short frame so that **I am able to eat more** without later **resorting** to dieting. *"In the final analysis, this eliminates the genetic argument for medical or morbid obesity, while recognizing that genes can certainly put us in a high-risk category for rapid and extreme weight gain."* (Apex)

With help, we can change our metabolic burn of calories no matter how much damage we have done to our bodies. Believe me, I damaged mine more than anyone I know, and I had genetic challenges as well.

**For many years I believed I was a prisoner of my genes, but clearly I WAS NOT!**

## The Dreaded Plateau

This is where most people quit, once they reach a plateau where they seem no longer capable of losing any weight no matter what they do. They may be keeping records and doing everything they have been told is absolutely right, yet the weight loss comes to a halt! I personally experienced several three-week long plateaus during the 18 month period in which I lost my weight. It was so devastating and anxiety-inducing that Al used to tease me and say he was thinking about tying me to the scale and throwing me in the Mississippi river! A little humor helps! Having the same struggles, we were able to tease each other.

To make a long story short, DON'T QUIT! Above all, please don't cut your calories and don't start running marathons. Remain on the calories laid out in your formula and continue to exercise. Do try and "manipulate" the exercise by changing it somewhat. Talk to your personal trainer about how to do this. Progression and manipulation of your exercise program is discussed in this chapter. If you start with "maximal" exercise (the way the weight loss challenge shows do on TV), then you have NO PLACE to go in the progression and manipulation of your exercise in order to ward off a plateau.

The bottom line is metabolism. Our bodies have some kind of well-explored but not completely understood regulatory mechanism that works to keep our energy (calorie) intake and output in balance. I now refer to the plateau as a "short-term metabolic adjustment." Water retention can also greatly contribute to actual weight gain or a plateau. It is a very complex matter and some of the resources on my resource page, if studied seriously, can help you on that.

If you persevere through the plateau IT WILL RE-ADJUST ITSELF. Also, remember that the closer you get to your goal, the slower the weight loss becomes. If you accept this concept, you will realize that you are nearing your final goal, and your perseverance will be blessed. Mine certainly was.

# CHAPTER FOUR

### *KEYWORDS FOR CHANGE*

*The mind can be changed!*

New habits can become automatic, just as bad habits got into your brain and they are automatic. This requires some focused work, but *well worth ultimately having your mind re-programmed forever*!

Don't ask God "Why, Why, Why?" Ask Him "What, what, what?" What do I do God…? Show me, guide me. I am ready to practice TRUTH!"

**Short-term vs. Lifelong Success.**

In regard to radical solutions and diets, including bariatric surgeries, if the solution turns out to accomplish rapid weight loss or "physician assisted starvation" we may not immediately **recognize the need to re-program our minds** with regard to food and/or exercise, and various lifestyle habits. This short-term success is, therefore, usually just that: short term! For the surgery patient, as post- op years increase, we will certainly notice the gradual increase in weight gain as we are able to have more food and have not yet adopted a *consistent* walking/exercise program. Unfortunately, when we arrive at this point we won't have the **safety net** of having done a lot of mental work and internal changes in attitude and habits, because until that moment arrived we did not have to, and we probably thought we would never have to. Simply said, the radical solution worked **too well** for too long. And it did not result in lifetime peace and maintenance.

## USE THE FOLLOWING KEYWORDS TO CHANGE YOUR BRAIN!

## THE SURGEON OPERATED ON YOUR STOMACH, NOT YOUR BRAIN!

### DELAY

Use DELAY whenever you are tempted. For example: before you buy that box of cookies, which you know doesn't need to be in your house, pray immediately and ask God to work with this focused tool of "delay." Say, "Jesus help me, I am using the word and the tool of delay against the enemy." You will find that with a deliberate delay from buying the cookies, of only 5-10 minutes, that God will actually remove the temptation *because He is blessing your obedience*. For a long time, you will have to use the "delay method" because of the years of stronghold from the enemy is this area. Speak the word DELAY out loud. Be ready to use it.

Set it in your brain. Pray for God to bless this tool. You will be **amazed,** *through your small five minute response to God, how incredible His response is to you!*

Let's go much deeper with this "delay" tool using Oswald Chambers'

> *"with focused attention and great care, you have to "work out" what God "works in" you. – not work to accomplish or earn "your own salvation," but work it*

*out so you will exhibit the evidence of a life based with determined, unshakable faith of the complete and perfect redemption of the Lord. As you do this, you do not bring an opposing will up against God's will – God's will is your will. ...The only thing to do with our barrier of stubbornness is to blow it up with "dynamite," and the **"dynamite" is obedience to the Holy Spirit.**[13]*

*Do not merely listen to the word, and so deceive yourselves; do what it says.*

**James 1:22 NIV**

*Mary tells the servers at the wedding "Do whatever He tells you."*

**John 2:5B NAB**

## CUES

Think about the "cues" you are receiving daily in regard to food. Are you confusing the cue to sleep or relax with a hunger cue? Are you confusing the cue for a good, filling balanced meal with the cue for a box of cookies? Are you confusing the cue for relaxing exercise time with the cue to eat when you are not even hungry? Are you confusing the cue for thirst with the need for food? *Recognize and define the real cues you that are receiving and don't be confused into exceeding your calorie boundaries with a false cue.*

Repeat these important words until this knowledge becomes automatic in your mind. For instance, for years I

---

[13] My Utmost for Your Highest Oswald Chambers

confused the cue of thirst with hunger. Now, it is automatic for me to recognize thirst immediately. I had to practice focused attention to this confusion for a while.

## FEAR

**2 Timothy 1:7** NIV "For *God has not given us the spirit of fear, but of love, of power, and of a sound mind.*" For people who have gained their weight back over and over, fear of failure once again keeps them captive. This is a **tool** that our enemy uses and we must remember that **fear is not of God.** Power and a sound mind can result from education in nutrition and exercise, but not from impatience promoted by the fast weight loss industry. I began to develop power and a sound mind through education at the medical school and continual study in textbooks while I attainted educational units over the years as a trainer. Let's go deeper with Oswald Chambers on fear:

> *...what are you fearing? Whatever it may be, you are not a coward about it – you are determined to face it, yet you still have a feeling of fear. When it seems that there is nothing and no one to help you, say to yourself, "But, the Lord is my helper this very moment, even in my present circumstance." Take hold of the Father's assurance, and then say with strong courage, "I will not fear." It does not matter what evil or wrong may be in our way, because "He Himself has said 'I will never leave you...'*[14]

---

[14] My Utmost for Your Highest

I remember **how fearful I was on long, repeated plateaus** and how much I just wanted to "starve myself" out of it and get there fast. But, I was studying the facts on metabolism, and I knew that God had educated me with the truth. Starving myself out of it would only hurt me in the long run……. I had to take hold of the Father's many assurances that He had given me *and not let fear stop me from moving forward using the whole truth of how God made us!*

## PANIC

Don't believe in the **scale.** Believe in the **program.** Believe in the **food records** that you have kept. Believe in the **walking** that you are doing. Focus on the program, because the scale often brings panic, which is where evil can do its work and cause you to you quit. Rest assured, when you feel panic, it is **not** of God. Focus on your new habits and keep records to have an "honest appraisal" of how you are doing over time. *This will keep you out of the "victim mentality" and your focus will be on improving your consistency in what is required, instead of on the scale.*

## DENIAL

Denial protects us at times. It can temporarily be a useful, powerful emotion. However, we eventually have to face the truth. *Face the fear and* **remove denial** *over the changes you should make.* Don't **convince** yourself that you are exercising and not losing weight, when the exercise is sporadic, not consistent; hey, you really **only walked twice** in the last four weeks!

Don't convince yourself that you are truly within your calorie boundaries just because you never touch a piece of white bread. You can be outside of the calorie ranges to lose and maintain weight even with the most "perfect" foods in the world. Keep the food and exercise records. Have a great desire to **really know** what has gone on in your body by keeping simple records, instead of falling into the "victim mentality" all the time.

Choosemyplate.gov and Weight Watchers teach you how to keep simple records, no more difficult than keeping your checkbook transactions. **Phone apps** are also great! My favorite one is livestrong.com… easy! If the **records show** that you have not made enough improvements, you can work on those. **Avoid denial at all costs.** It has hurt you long enough. Have a goal of getting back into those smaller clothes in your closet, instead of not facing that they just don't fit, denying the reason you bought new clothes is because you were two sizes larger than last year. (I guess you can tell how long I practiced denial!). Face the facts and practice the solutions! Don't be the spouse who says to your partner, "You are supposed to love me no matter what"! What you are *really saying is,* "Don't criticize me about all this weight which I don't want to work on, no matter how it hurts our relationship in numerous ways." If you are in denial about the last time you had sex because you are ashamed of your body and you don't "feel sexy" for your spouse because of all this fat, then you *are hurting your spouse and* **you are the one** *out of biblical guidelines*!

You are the one who is **not** acting as if you love your spouse "no matter what." You are the one who has to do something. (We are not talking about the unreasonable spouse who wants much more than a *healthy weight* for you and is unhappy that you do not look like you did before you had children.)

### IMPATIENCE "WAITING, WAITING, WAITING"

The fruits of the spirit are listed in **Galatians 5:22.** Patience is one of them. **Patience is very hard to adopt** when we are given **fast fixes on a platter**, so to speak, from people we **trust.** But, impatience does not give us a lifelong, permanent solution in any specific area of our lives. We cannot use impatience with raising children, in our marital relationships, meeting our financial needs and goals, or achieving an education. Success in these areas always requires long, hard, detailed and dedicated work.

> *Developing patience also helps to define short term goals which will gradually lead us to our long term destination. Focus on the daily journey and weekly goals, not on how long it will take to get there. Keep doing this God's way because God's Timing is Perfect.*
> **Deeper with Oswald Chambers:**

*"If our hopes seem to be experiencing disappointment right now, it simply means that they are being purified. Every hope or dream of the human mind will be fulfilled if it is noble and of God.* ***But one of the greatest stresses in life is the stress of waiting on God.*** *He brings fulfillment, "because you have kept my commandment to persevere...."*[15]

---

[15] My Utmost for Your Highest

*(Rev. 3:10)*17

I finally realized that waiting is *not a waste of time* when you are a growing Christian. You may be going through a purging process that will not be lifted until *God's work in your heart is complete*. Repeat, repeat, repeat: God's timing is perfect. When the wait feels impossible, I focus on building patience and my relationship with Christ, rather than fretting, fretting, fretting, which is nothing more than a waste of time and a distraction from the task at hand.

## SKILL POWER, NOT WILLPOWER

Skill power comes from studying the right educational material for nutrition and exercise. My resource page will help you develop this. Many of my bullet tips, throughout this book, are "skill powers" to be developed. After you study and develop many of these new skills, and you feel you are not doing well, ask yourself: have you really worked hard on all the "skill powers" you have learned? These skill powers REPLACE THE NEED for willpower, which most obese people do not have.

*Forget trying to develop will power, and start working harder on skill power.*

After all this time, I **still do not possess that "nail biting, teeth clenching, weeping" willpower needed to erase or manage obsessive habits.** I must continue to work very hard on skill powers that have given me much greater success against habitual problems. I still occasionally experience fleeting moments of weakness depending on how fabulous Satan's attacks are, but I have definitely been set free from the habitual problems which used to enslave me. What exactly is enslavement? This is when other areas of our lives and relationships are negatively affected by our obsessive behavior and where we are powerless to overcome it no matter how destructive its effects.

I would like to ask you this question: How many times have you tried **willpower**? How many times have you failed using that alone? Stop repeating insanity and try working on more **skill power** and join me in peaceful, lifetime weight maintenance! Many teach that insanity is doing the same thing over and over and expecting different results!

Also, sheer will power sometimes creates pride, arrogance, and strong criticism and opinions of others toward those who are still in this awful struggle. The spirit of God sets us free *forever*, (by working on and learning skill powers in all areas of life.) This slow, hard work normally creates humility, gratitude and compassion for others, instead of arrogant criticism.

## SELF CONTROL

This is different than self-discipline in my opinion. I will explain that using an example later in this paragraph. Self-control is listed as one of the **fruits of the spirit in Galatians 5:17.** In the area that we are speaking, in controlling our food intake , my opinion is that this self-control for us follows on the heels of "skill power," **instead of the teeth clenching "will power"** that most of us cannot maintain over time.

For instance, one of my skill powers is making certain to slice a few oranges every morning and have them waiting for me in the fridge. Every time I open the refrigerator door to satisfy my oral craving I see them. There are times when I think, oh, it is almost bedtime… I feel really hungry…. and I am tempted to gorge on a 300 calorie bowl of cereal, when I only have 60 calories left in my daily allowance. When *the fruit of self-control is exercised or comes into play,* I will go in and gorge on that 60 calorie orange and love it! After I eat it, I am satisfied. This reaction is based on the years of skill power that I have practiced. It is not even very often that this "self-control" is needed, but sometimes it is, usually when I am tired or stressed. There is a sweet, sweet harvest and lasting satisfaction that comes from using a bit of self-control, as opposed to how most of us with these problems perceive willpower. FOR SURGERY PATIENTS: My goodness….. you can "push back from that food serving so much EASIER than other people…. Recognize that you are full and satisfied sooner than others who do not have this edge! PRACTICE LIFELONG GRATITUDE for the EDGE this SURGERY gives you in self-control! IT WILL GIVE YOU AN EDGE LIFELONG, but **not like in the early days** of your surgery. **Use the early days and years** of the surgery to **change your brain** with new habits! Those people who have never had really severe problems and strongholds with this problem just love to use the word "self-discipline" toward us. They don't understand that this self- discipline has been stolen from us in innocent childhood, or slowly later in life. We must "learn" this again and it is a long road up. But, we can do it!

## EUPHORIA AND TRANSFER ADDICTION

The emotion of euphoria comes first with a large weight loss. Beware of it! It is so good to finally be free from your biggest enemy, yourself! Euphoria is fine for a month or so but it is **not a helpful emotion** to have for a long time. It prevents us from truly facing the hard work at hand and in any case, it is not "real". It also helps to create for some people just another compulsive behavior right away, such as promiscuity, alcoholism, arrogance, etc. Pray that God will balance you out emotionally, but euphoria is not a good balance. For those of us with addictive food disorders, "transfer addiction" is common and we must be *aware* of it to avoid it. We simply go from one addiction to another. For example, I have seen alcoholics get rid of their addictive behavior, but immediately use food in excess and are a hundred pounds overweight within five years. One problem is as bad as another! Euphoria long term can contribute to this.

## ARMOR

Do not neglect your "closet time" with God. This means a quiet time with God on a daily basis, preferably in the mornings before your daily challenges, even if it is in the car during your commute, presenting to God your thanks, intercession for others, and all of your needs, no matter how small. Study **Philippians 4:6-7**. Read and rely on God "talking to you" through Psalms and other Bible scriptures.

Have a specific prayer time each and every day. *Expect* to have arrows thrown at you! (Read and absorb **Ephesians Chapter Six** in the New Testament…..read this often.) The arrows will not "penetrate" if your armor is on! Put your armor on daily. Soldiers would not go out even one day without their armor. Use your commute time in the car or delete a TV show to protect yourself by having God's armor always in place! You will eventually treasure and *look forward* to this as you see God's BEST resolutions in your life. Do not **underestimate** the complexity and cleverness of the evil forces in this world. Do not underestimate the true answer God has given you to fight these forces successfully. This is a daily battle. The least bit of overconfidence in your own strength, without God's resources, can lead you to much suffering. It is much easier to suffer for doing right than to withstand the suffering which follows when we do wrong. I have learned this the hard way. *When we start each day with God's resources, we will slowly prevail toward godly habits!*

**Ephesians 6: 16, 17, 18 NAB** "In ALL circumstances hold faith as a shield, to quench all the flaming arrows of the evil one. And take the helmet of salvation and the sword of the Spirit, which is the Word of God. With every prayer and request, pray at all times in the Spirit, and stay alert in this with all perseverance, and intercession for all the saints."

Do you have your armor on? The Shield, the Helmet, the Sword, and Prayer???

## "THOSE WHO FAIL TO PLAN, PLAN TO FAIL"

On my resource page you will find a healthy eating **plan** that you can live with that is not a fast fix. There will be one that will match your own personality. Just eating and exercising healthy creates less of these psychological urges.

However, many times in my life I was on a healthy eating plan and ultimately these urges took over, so it is *only one keyword* among many others that you will need. Designing my own plan within pleasant and reasonably healthy boundaries is what works for me. Within this concept you can include surgery restrictions, but pray about what the clinics tell you. They are very; very, very "dieting" oriented which can lead to a backfire for you!

## YOKE

When we take care of a problem *without following all the biblical guidelines*, the yoke becomes so much more difficult and a cycle of failure and *more difficulty* always results, becoming like a large weight around your neck. This is not just with fast weight loss and the eventual problems it causes, but with money, relationships, and other important issues we face in life. The Bible guidelines are practical and work! I understand now about "God's yoke" being easy. I have also been stubborn in other areas and had to find out that *God's way is always easier than my way.*

## DESIRE

There must be a personal, magnificent desire to overcome any addiction or severe problem. We have all have seen the "interventions" for alcohol and drug abuse on TV. In some of the stories, the intervention teams and family are the *only ones* with this great desire. They have intervened before any sincere desire is expressed from the addicted party. The great desire to overcome an addiction or a bad habit, or just to make a good new habit, must come from the person himself. God can do this for you. **What we can <u>tolerate</u> is not something we can overcome!** I cannot tolerate obesity for myself. This is not about discrimination, but about my health and energy!

## CONDEMNATION OR CONVICTION?

In **Galatians Chapter Three**, it states that we grow in Christ-like character, one step at a time, by getting into stride with God's grace and mercy, not by law or legalism. Others may impose *legalism* on you in food and exercise, but God will not. God knows better than anyone through what manner a Christian has developed the stronghold of food and exercise problems, (and sometimes it has been through someone else's legalism and pride over their own self- discipline about food and exercise choices.) God knows you and still loves you. He is able to *love* you into slowly changing this area of weakness and bondage in your life. He will help you to tackle one area at a time.

The following is the scripture that often "fell open" in my Bible for over thirty years in regard to my repeated failure over this problem.

> *This high priest (Jesus) of ours understands our weaknesses, since he had the same temptations that we do, though he never once gave way to them and sinned. So let us come boldly to the very throne of God, and stay there to receive his mercy and his grace, to help us in our times of need.*
>
> **(Hebrews 4: 15-16)**

## INSTANT GRATIFICATION

Ask yourself why you are about to consume food outside of your boundaries for instant gratification. Is it because of stress, loneliness, fatigue, depression, boredom, or because you're in a hurry? Instant gratification can turn into years of misery as you may already know.

## DEPRIVATION

I believe the greatest lesson God can teach you in the area of food is to teach you "no deprivation." For example, if you have an incredible craving for a candy bar that will not go away using the "tool of delay I mentioned," then **get half** of a candy bar, or even just *one* candy bar, and **count** it in your food records, and *enjoy* it slowly. **Readjust** your calories at night to a large vegetarian meal, etc. God will help you not to struggle anymore. Our demons love to make you fail 159 times because you make a **practice** of losing and maintaining weight by using severe deprivation. I no longer do that. I estimate my liberal calorie allotment daily and find a way to "cheat" within it. There are no magic foods and there are no bad foods. Study my resource page. It will educate you on nourishment for your body which is so important, but will not tell you "never to cheat." I consider surgery restrictions of course.

**Nourish** your body with the appropriate balance of protein, carbs, and fats in a good meal. You will be amazed how this will **automatically** reduce your need to eat too many rich or processed foods.

## RUSHING

Work on your schedule so that you do not always feel rushed. As you develop simplification at different stages of your life, you will come to recognize how "rushing" creates overeating and bad choices. I suggest that you work and pray on this "rushing" thing way before you work on food tips and exercise tips in Chapter Seven.

Believe me; in looking at my life over these last forty five years, I experienced all the "stages." I was super Mom, super wife, and super church member, experienced financial problems, made personal mistakes, and lived in a bad marriage for twelve years of the 30 year marriage. (Al changed, ha-ha! Well, he changed first!)

I now see many, many areas that I could have totally simplified during any one of these life stages. I still look back and see that I could have erased some of the "hurried" lifestyle with small children. I could have worked harder at "simplifying" life in any of those stages, and paid more attention to the things I needed to do to overcome food and exercise problems. Only you and God can work on that, and believe me, He will lead you. God knows better than you that a host of things need to be changed in your life in order to succeed 100% with **permanent** weight loss. One thing is certain: He wants you off this ridiculous dieting madness and it is a lie that you have to diet forever!

## HUNGER

Eat as soon as possible when you find that you are getting really hungry. Do not reach the point of starving before you take the time to eat, even if it means having a healthy snack before you can get to a meal. This requires some planning, perhaps having food with you. I used low fat peanut butter wheat crackers which made me feel good and satisfied, but any healthy snack will do, preferably one which also contains protein, fat, and carbs. The calories are noted on the package of these crackers, so I was able to figure them into my daily calorie allowance. I also carry along some quartered oranges when I am at work and need a quick snack to keep me from getting too hungry before my next meal. The fiber in this snack fills you, despite the lack of protein and fat. Find your own plan and tricks and stick to it. Also recognize if it is real hunger or something else in "HALT" that needs to be addressed in another way, for instance, by using the "DELAY" method. (HALT is an acronym for "hungry, angry, lonely, and tired).

## ANGER AND DEPRESSION

These problems may result from present or past relationships/ experiences or they could be over financial problems, or an unexpected loss or radical change of any type. Use the Four P's: prayer, preparation, planning, and patience to help you combat anger and depression. Remember, even a good psychiatrist never learns everything about you and knows far less than God does in any event. God's mercy and understanding of you is beyond your imagination! God will direct you as to how to eradicate anger and depression from your life. He may lead you to the right medication if it is a physical problem. **Remember that regular aerobic exercise greatly helps with mood levels (the good mood levels of beta endorphins are raised and the stress hormone of cortisol levels are reduced).**

## LONELINESS

I never thought this would happen for me. Loneliness for too many people results in addictive behavior such as food addiction, alcoholism, and whatever the "addiction of choice" might be.

Never had I experienced true loneliness in my life until my husband of thirty years died unexpectedly when I was forty-nine and a half years old. Al was fifty-two when he died. The year before his death, our last child had left the nest. My oldest child had left the nest three years earlier. The three of them had been the focus of my whole life at home for *three decades!* I thank God that I at least I had my new work as a trainer in place before Al's passing. Despite that, the loneliness was unreal! I did not purposely think about it and focused on staying very busy throughout the day, determined not to indulge in self-pity for the sake of my blossoming children in their young adult years. I remained productive and busy as a personal trainer and in church life.

Despite my productive lifestyle, **the loneliness pressed against me like a freight train.** Thank God that he was long-suffering with me; forgiving and merciful when two years later I sought the wrong solutions with male company and flavored cigars (yes, can you believe it?)

God's "freight train" of love pressed against me too, and mercifully, the victory was His! I do not believe that anyone can truly empathize with this type of loneliness unless he has experienced it firsthand. Loneliness is different than being alone. Being alone is something that I have always enjoyed and great power comes from solitude on a regular basis. But *true loneliness* is torture, like solitary confinement in prison, and it *even* occurs with loved ones and friends around and sometimes that is even the worst. I never expected a continual "ache" like this and I used the wrong methods, out of desperation, to address it. Since 2006 God has done a miracle of causing me to know that loneliness will pass, and it is now very short term.

## FATIGUE

Work hard to protect your rest and sleep. If you have sleep apnea, do all you can to correct this as it will rob you of needed energy. Be *proactive in finding the time to rest instead of pushing yourself. When you are tired you are more prone to feel depressed, to be in a hurry, and to be lazy in choosing the right foods.* You will definitely not feel like all the preparation needed for home meals like plenty of cut up fresh veggies. You also won't feel like getting the exercise you need. Don't underestimate the role that being overly-tired plays in your struggle with maintaining a healthy weight. If you have a problem with sleep, pray for God to help you with this and be pro-active in the course God gives you to pursue a resolution. On the other hand, don't underestimate the energy and relief from tiredness that a good walking program and a balanced menu will give you! When exhausted, try ten minutes of walking and if your energy level does not rise up noticeably, you probably really need to rest! Rarely, however, have I gone home after ten minutes of walking because I got the blood pumping and raised my energy level! It also cleared my head. God made us like this!

## PERFECTIONISM

Perfectionism causes stress and an unnecessarily complicated lifestyle. It robs many people of the time to exercise regularly, to keep the house food-proofed or food friendly consistently, and to prepare healthy meals. I have seen this with many people who are overweight, most especially with a number of my clients as I have gotten to know them well. Pray about which areas of your life that you can "let go of" in practicing perfectionism. It is good to be detailed and get things done right, *but please examine if this is affecting your time to stay healthy.*

## PROGRESS AND REGRESS

While you go about **learning** new behavioral patterns, you will inevitably regress at times. When you do, immediately recognize how well you have progressed in other areas. Give yourself *time* to anchor your new skills. Do not allow yourself to fall into self- condemnation over any area of regression, or depression will step in and create a *stronghold*. Identify where you may need to *hold off* in progressing. Remember that God is not in a hurry to *get you all the way there to your healthy weight goal*, even though a bad habit that still exists will eventually need to go. God is much more interested in developing the "workman" than the final work. Remembering this will help you to remain patient for the final victory! God is patient!

> *"God will perfect and accomplish that which concerneth you."*
>
> **Psalm 138:8 NKJV**

I encourage you to become anchored in **one new level of progress at a time.** God wants you totally anchored there *first*. Once you have a 100% comfort level in that one specific area, ask God which new area you can comfortably work on. He is not in a hurry to go to the next level of weeding out these deeply rooted problems in your life and in your mind. Each time you have regressed momentarily, learn to praise God for all the stages of progression He has already given you victory in!

At times you will KNOW that you have reached a level of success in one area, you will feel it and without a doubt know that you are where you need to be. Repeat to yourself, "Don't regress… you have achieved a solid rock anchor in this area," claim your victory and move forward….and begin to work on a new area to reclaim. You have won one battle and can proceed to the next troop of "enemy soldiers!"

David wrote: **Psalm 18:29** *"For it is by my God that I have run through a troop of enemy soldiers and it is by my God that I have leaped over a tall wall."* And wow this is a tall wall!

## PATIENCE

I also used the word "impatience" earlier. This book addresses fast weight loss and how America has been captured by that method primarily because of our problems with patience! I will beat this dead horse once more! Of course, patience is a keyword and was my first keyword I used as God lovingly knocked me in the head with it in 1996.

Waiting on a complete weight loss, slowly, is difficult, but it is best.

### The Ultimate Race, by Charles Stanley

> *"Throughout the 26.2 mile run, a marathon runner's body goes through many changes. He must fight the inclination to move too fast early in the race. He must overcome muscle cramps and blisters. He must ignore the whispering voice mid-way through that says, "You've already done a great job. Everyone is impressed that you even got this far. Why don't you just quit now?"*
> 
> *With every step, the runner reaffirms his decision to keep going, to move closer and closer to the finish line. His eye is on the goal, and he will not be distracted or denied. This is endurance.*

*To endure does not mean to sit back, take it easy, or look for a way out. Nor does the word mean to casually accept a setback and quit the race early. Rather, it is the sense of "staying power." This involves the initiative to do whatever it takes to win – like pushing through obstacles and throwing off any hindrances, one step at a time, as you keep moving. In hardships, trials, and heartaches, endurance means you won't quit until you have achieved victory.*

*This is the image we should keep in mind as we read the challenge to "lay aside every encumbrance... (and) run with endurance the race that is set before us."*

*Whatever it takes, Lord, I'm going to get there. I will not give up. I will not step off your path until you've brought me to the finish line."*

# CHAPTER FIVE

## *DISCOVER A LOVE FOR MOVEMENT AT ANY AGE!*

*There was a time when I dreaded walking to the mailbox; now I have fun physical hobbies which I do as second nature to me that involve jumping, bending, twisting, rowing, and moving rapidly. Change your focus to agility and health, not on how you look.*

**So how did I get from A to Z, from severe obesity to a level of fitness that allows me to live a fully active and joyful life?**

Although I had enjoyed walking in the past, I was never consistent over time. I was under the illusion that if I walked I would lose weight very efficiently and when this didn't happen, I would inevitably give up.

I now understand that if you are consuming too many calories you will not lose weight, **even** if you walk consistently. What failed to register with me at the time was that while walking I **had at least stopped gaining weight.**

*Maintenance is a victory, at any weight, especially when you are enjoying food.*

Walking consistently, **40 minutes 5 days weekly**, was just an *obligation* for a long time. It was only about making the weight come off while allowing myself a generous amount of calories for my size, instead of starving myself, which had never worked for long. It was about raising my metabolism instead of damaging it once again. It was an obligation and a sacrifice I felt I had to make for myself and my family, but it wasn't fun.

Slowly, as I kept it up, embracing **patience** as my friend, and **knowing** that I was obeying God, **surprisingly,** *the obligation gradually turned to **enjoyment**!* As I walked for forty minutes, five days a week, I prayed. I listened to motivational Christian music in a fanny pack around my waist. The music became my walking partner! It was more dependable than a human partner, and the hour also doubled as devotional time. I listened to God and He listened to me. I began to look forward to the stress relief of the music and to the surge of energy that I always felt afterwards.

**STRESS RELIEF**. I know that after a long day of work, few of us feel motivated to put on exercise clothes and go out for a power walk, and there were a couple of nights when ten minutes into my walk I knew I was too tired to go on, so I returned home to rest and retire early. It is good to listen to your body so that you don't risk injury, and you should never push yourself when, for whatever reason, you are really too exhausted to do a forty minute walk. **However, it is a physiological fact that movement makes the blood rush through your body quickly and gives you a boost of energy, something we all welcome after a long work day. Once you experience this a few times, you won't forget it! It is also a physiological fact that aerobic exercise raises the beta-endorphin levels and reduces cortisol levels. Once you**

**identify and experience this, you will want to do it for stress relief only!**

God always provides the time for something that is truly in biblical guidelines.

Continuing my walking routine at night gradually became very difficult to maintain after a long day of work. Al lived in New York City at that time on assignment from IBM, his last year to work before he became too sick. I had errands to do at night and missed Al's help. I prayed that God would help me find a solution. I prayed about asking the physician I was working for at the time to give me an hour and 15 minutes for lunch instead of just an hour. I promised to stay an extra 15 minutes at the end of the day. This way I could enjoy a full exercise program at lunch, eat a can of Healthy Choice Soup at my desk, and "steal" an hour out of my workday for exercise. He said yes! Praise God!

Exercise was no longer an obligation, but something that I looked forward to as the highlight of my day. It slowly transformed into "play", and my whole attitude changed. It is still the highlight of my day. For many years now my life has been about enjoying food and many calories (guilt-free, the best kind!), while achieving weight maintenance, relieving daily stress, raising my mood level, and finding fun, outdoor hobbies to share with my family and friends.

At the **end of my exercise time,** I always think, **"I can't wait until tomorrow so I can do this all over again!"** I doubt this would ever happen to weight loss challenge contestants on TV. It is reported that most of them do not stay with their program for a lifetime. It is reported that 70% have regained their weight. **If this is not the way you feel after your exercise routine, if instead you are thinking, "Oh no, not again tomorrow," you are probably doing too much, too soon.**

*Moderation in exercise* can lead to <u>lifetime</u> frequency, consistency, and enjoyment. Unless you are competing in high- level sports, exercise should not be work for you, but a time of play.

**If you have a history of "stopping and starting" then ask yourself if you did too much, too soon.**

**How to Re-discover Play and Remembering My Husband, Al.**

*We would all rather play than work; one is an obligation, the other is pure joy.*

I remember one night while I walked seeing the outline of my shadow in the street lights. There was a small, shapely, slender silhouette that I didn't at first recognize. Honestly, I did not realize that it was me! I continued to walk and thought to myself, "I wonder if I can run?" I had not picked up my feet to run since I was 18 years old and played tennis. Hesitatingly, I began a slow jog. I picked up the pace a bit, although it was a strange feeling after so many years of being nailed to the ground by my weight. As I neared our house I began to sob like a baby. I could not believe that I was running! I entered the front door of the house, sobbing loudly. Al came as fast as he could into the foyer. He thought that I had been hurt. *I looked straight at him and exclaimed, "Al, I ran."* He looked at me and smiled, with tears in his eyes. No one else could have understood the tremendous significance of those words. We said nothing more, but just held each other. As I write these years after his death, I remember his cute face so clearly standing in that foyer, and smiling at me! He was so proud of me! That night was FUN.... PLAY..... NOT EXERCISE!

## Don't Be Afraid of Gyms!

In 1995, I was living in that same suburban neighborhood where I first jogged. We had access to a three-mile circle outside my front door. There was a walking lane as well as a large and popular athletic club in the area. I never would have dreamed of going to the club as I assumed everyone who belonged must look like Suzie Body Builder or Bikini Suzie! I couldn't ever imagine walking through the front door, much less signing up for a membership. This was the large gym that eventually hired me as a trainer. For years, before my husband died, I worked a steady fifty-hour week helping people in my former situation, and I saw very few Suzie's there. Don't ever assume that only extremely fit, trim people have athletic club memberships. I see all types at the club, and everyone has his own reason for being there. Don't hesitate to walk through those doors; someone like me with my history might be waiting for you on the other side!

All this may sound like discipline, but I was having FUN, and as children know, fun does not require discipline or willpower. I was no longer Pam Harrelson alone on the road in the dark... I was Pamster the Great! It was not the old me, forcing myself to fulfill an obligation. I was now a child at play, just as God had created me.

Although my exercise mode and routine has been adjusted over time for my age and lifestyle, I am **still a child at play**. This can happen to you!

### How I Discovered New Hobbies

I sold the house three years after Al died and decided to create a new life all my own, in essence, a new "Pam Harrelson." This would be an active life and I prayed that I would find the right place to live in order to promote a new and active lifestyle. My two requirements were that there be no mortgage and there would be "built-in" physical activity to keep me motivated to move as I became older. When I discovered the condo complex I knew almost immediately that God had sent me to the right place. I would have pitched a tent here had there not been an available condo! There are only seven other owners, all single, all about the same age, so I don't have to go far to find companionship. Just yesterday we rode the bike trace to a restaurant one hour away and even did some "dirt biking" on some paths. I felt like a child! The residents ten years younger than myself always invite me for their bike rides!

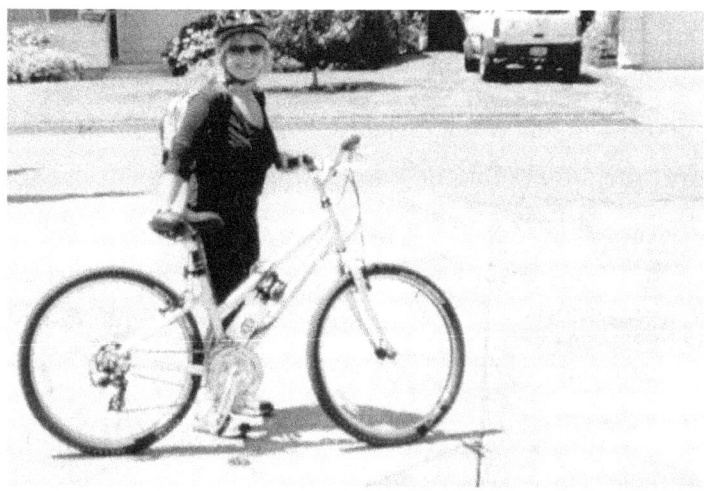

*Biking in summer heat in my late 50's.*

Please notice my agility in the following story details of my Kayak. Desire this agility for yourself! It is not too late. You **can get that old friend back** who had more character, greater energy and more agility!

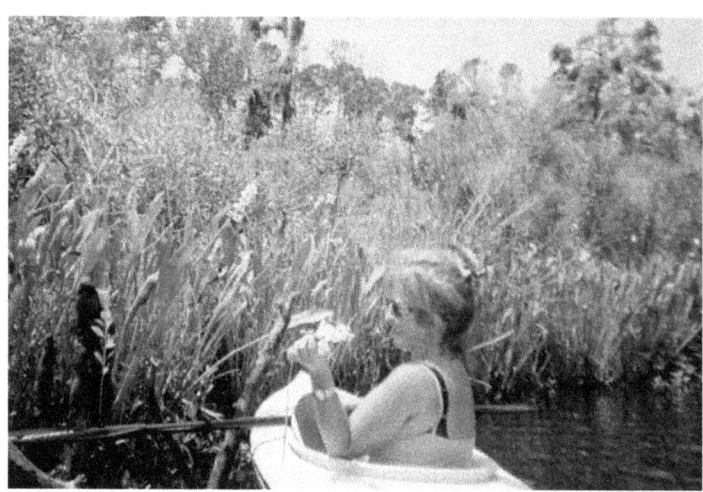

Yesterday I went out my back door to wash my three-seater Sea- Doo. It sits on a floating dock on my boat slip, just yards from my back porch. My two-seater kayak rests beside it, easily mountable from the floating dock. I grabbed the hose and power-washed the Sea-Doo. Then I jumped down onto the floating dock from the finger pier, and balanced myself around the small edge of the floating dock which the ski sits on. I climbed back and forth over my Sea-Doo, polishing and scrubbing until it shined. When I was done I hopped on my bike and rode down to the library, checked out some books, packed them in my little bike basket and headed home.

I read a bit, then watched some news on TV while I ate a tomato sandwich with some low fat cheese and a bag of low fat 100 calories chips for something crunchy. I topped it off with an orange, but then I had a cookie "attack" so went to my neighbor Jim's and got one of his cookies! I have "skill power" but still no will power; therefore, if a sack of cookies were in the house I might possibly eat them all under stress! Using some "skill power," I made sure to fill up on healthy food before getting the cookie, so that just one would satisfy my sweet tooth.

Then, I decided to paddle in the kayak for a while. I pulled the heavy kayak close to the edge of the water, lifted up the end of it, and threw it into the water. It landed right beside the floating dock and Sea- Doo. If you aren't careful getting into the kayak, you can tip over into the bayou, so I carefully put one foot close to the seat and got into a "squat" position before putting the other foot in. It is necessary to sit down immediately once your full weight is in the kayak, and this requires agility and balance. Before I was this careful, of course, I did flip over and fall into the bayou once.

That was the day I discovered how fast I can move! Our bayou has large turtles and small to medium-sized alligators in it, and, of course, there are the snakes. Needless to say, we don't voluntarily swim in the bayou! On the day I fell in, I found out I could shoot up out of the water like a living bullet and land rapidly right on the top of the dock! I didn't exactly relish the thought of a gator bite or having my toes nibbled by snapping turtles. I quickly learned to get in and out of my kayak without further incident.

**Don't miss the following sad story of a sweet, sad daddy on the river. If I can't motivate you to have the surgery or to lose the weight, maybe he can!**

When I was a mere fifty-two years old I was spending a beautiful sunny day with a good friend on jet skis on the nearby river. In the most crowded section of the river, where caution was needed to avoid collisions with the many boats and Jet Skis on the water that day, we saw a father and his young daughter floating in the water beside their turned over Jet Ski.

It is relatively easy to climb on top of a submerged Jet Ski and flip it back over. The directions for this maneuver are always written on the back of the Jet Ski. It is very important to do this quickly so that you can remount it from the back and **get out of the crowded water way.**

My friend and I stopped because there seemed to be no effort from the father to turn the ski over and get his daughter quickly to safety. We could only see their heads bobbing in the water so it would have been easy to overlook them. My friend, Mike, a tall lanky guy and very fit for fifty-two, pulled up close to the man and asked if he knew how to turn the ski over. When he said no, Mike agilely jumped into the water, put one arm over the top of the ski and quickly flipped it over. Then he crawled back onto his own Ski. We started to take off, until we noticed that the man made no move to mount his Ski. At that time, the little girl was picked up in a boat by what appeared to be family or friends. The man was left behind in the water, but strangely still made no attempt to get back on the Ski, so we turned around and went back to see if there was a problem. Mike asked him if he knew how to mount it. We figured he had borrowed it and really knew nothing about it. He said no. We instructed him but he still made no attempt. Finally, Mike offered to tow the Ski to the nearby dock with the man hanging onto the end. Afterward, we drove off, and looking back over our shoulders we watched as the young father emerged from the water, slowly pulling him up by the dock ladder. He probably weighed between 350 and 400 pounds.

As we watched him climb the ladder, the "mystery" was solved.

He did not have a heavy face or double chin so we could not tell previously that he was morbidly obese. Mike and I were both close to tears as we watched him struggle to slowly climb the ladder.

Because of his morbid obesity, a young father who had only wanted to give his daughter a fun day on the river was unable to rescue her from harm in an unexpected emergency. In his embarrassment over his physical condition, he could not even tell us why he wouldn't even attempt to mount the Sea-Doo.

*My heart was breaking. I felt so grateful for my own agility, mobility, and health, but I* had been where he was and knew firsthand how disappointed in himself, how ashamed and embarrassed he was probably feeling at that moment.

I wanted to give him the "book" that was only in my heart and in my mind at that time, a book that would motivate people to enjoy mobility and good health, one that would take the focus off of the way we look, and put it back on the quality of life we should all be able to enjoy for the longest possible time.

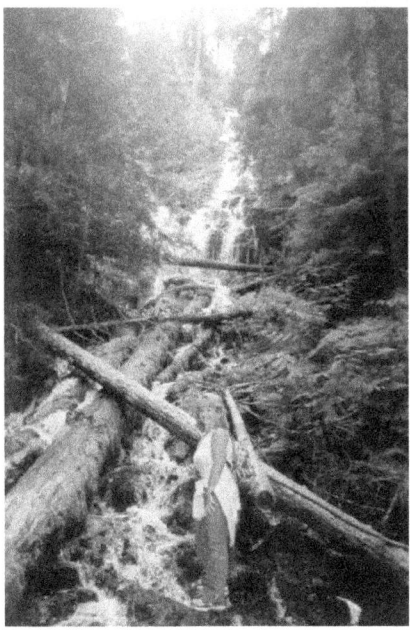

*Hiking in Oregon – 300 feet down at Proxy Falls! Age 52.*

I thought about the man later that night as I had a quiet time with the Lord. I prayed that the difficult moment he had on the water that day might motivate him to do something about his situation before it was too late.

**You don't have to run or push yourself to abnormal limits: If you get injured, you can't do anything! If you dread it, you will eventually do NOTHING!**

I lost my weight walking, and eventually went to a slow jog (Kinesiology experts say that duration, with an active but safe training heart rate, is good for weight loss, but that *intensity with less time* is required for weight maintenance.) Although I was not much of a runner I always felt like an "eagle" on my slow jogs. Perhaps because I had been immobile for so long, I often felt like I was flying! I loved the feeling of being in control of my body as I jogged along, and got the same "runner's high" that a **real runner** does as my adrenaline kicked in. I asked my daughter how I looked when I ran, as she saw me one day trotting along. I told her I felt like an eagle or a deer. She stuffed up some giggles and tried hard not to laugh. I asked her what was so funny. She said, "Mom, you look great running, but ….you look more like a little hamster on a treadmill because you are so tiny!" We both laughed hard, and after that she nicknamed me "Pamster." I told some clients at the club and from then on a few called me Pamster. I told Al and he said I looked like a little red-headed crawfish when I ran! Anyway, I still feel like an eagle or, at least, like "Pamster the Great" when I jog!

Many times, on the way home from an inspiring run, I would say this scripture out loud:

*Do you not know? Have you not heard? The Lord is the everlasting God, the Creator of the ends of the earth. He will not grow tired or weary, and his understanding no one can fathom. He gives strength to the weary and increases the power of the weak. Even youths grow tired and weary, and young men stumble and fall; but those who hope in the Lord will renew their strength. They will soar on wings like eagles; they will run and not grow weary, they will walk and not be faint.*

**Isaiah 40:28-31 NIV**

**Sometimes changes and transitions in life cause us to forget established exercise habits. DON'T DO THAT!**

My jogs at 4:30 in the morning before going to my work as a trainer at a large gym fell away after I took semi-retirement.

Whenever I have a **significant change** in my life, I try and make sure to post notes all around the house to remind myself as to when my new "formal" exercise time will be. I can't afford to give myself excuses and fall into old patterns of being sedentary. The exercise and active hobbies are stress-reducers and also distractions from eating out of boredom. When I'm restless, I practice one of my new active hobbies. But my "formal" exercise time has to be scheduled, no excuses allowed.

My new formal time is about 8:30 a.m. On four weekday mornings, which fits in better with my new, more relaxed schedule. My new exercise, at an older age, is biking. I bike the

Trace at a fast pace and go up the path to the Lake. I ride along Lakeshore drive and enjoy the tranquility of the water. I sprint a bit, and then go back to a slower pace. I pray the entire time and love that treasured time between the Lord and me outdoors in His wonderful creation.

In semi-retirement, I train just a few clients at a large athletic club and at my home gym. I lift light weights at home using my expertise from training. I used to lift heavy weights, but much has changed after menopause. I am still lifting enough to stay toned and to keep my bone density from worsening.

My present exercise time would still be considered moderate, consisting of about three hours of biking a week and about an hour of weights per week. This formal exercise is all I need to maintain my weight, with no "dieting," as long as I keep a daily approximate estimate of my 1500 calories. No foods or treats are considered "forbidden." I punished myself long enough. I consume a wide variety of good food, and some light "cheats," all within my calorie boundaries. I take in 1500 and burn up 1500, on a "7 day average," and maintain my weight in this manner. I am thankful to say that I have not been on a weight loss diet in many years.

My new hobbies on the water do not burn a lot of calories, but they add to the general calorie burn that I have. Taking care of my new pontoon boat, which I keep in the water, requires a lot of agility and a lot of energy. I have to jump into a five foot hole where the battery and motor is and I am only five feet tall. I must pull myself up out of the hole to get back into the boat! Certainly these hobbies burn more calories than the hobbies I once practiced, that is, TV, movies, and eating out! The paddling on the kayak is also a great stress reliever.

*The tranquility of the silent waterways is always pulling me to get outdoors just as food and a sedentary lifestyle used to pull me indoors. I have found play, fun, and joy with my new habits. They do not involve "discipline" in any way, shape, or form. Believe me: you can make this happen in your own life, one step at a time. Search for new hobbies to pull you away from bad ones!*

You are hearing someone talk to you who was sedentary for decades and who has been practicing this new lifestyle for decades. **Please know that God can work in your life to enable you to live a more active and healthy lifestyle that does not have to be competitive or punishing.** Pray about this, and then **do something to make it happen. God will <u>run to you</u> if you take the first steps! TRY IT!**

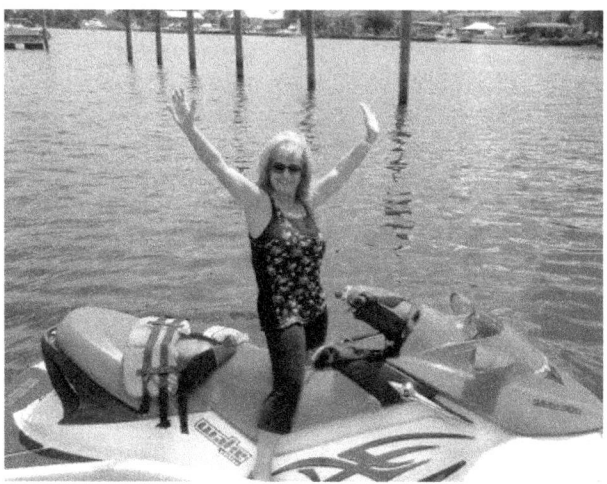

*Age 62*

Is exercise fun and active hobbies fun? Yes, it is fun, especially if you don't call it "exercise!" It is PLAY and in my case, the discovery of the joy of movement in middle age is the result of many prayed-over decisions to change my lifestyle from a sedentary to an active one.

# CHAPTER SIX

## *PERSONAL TRAINING FROM MY PERSPECTIVE*

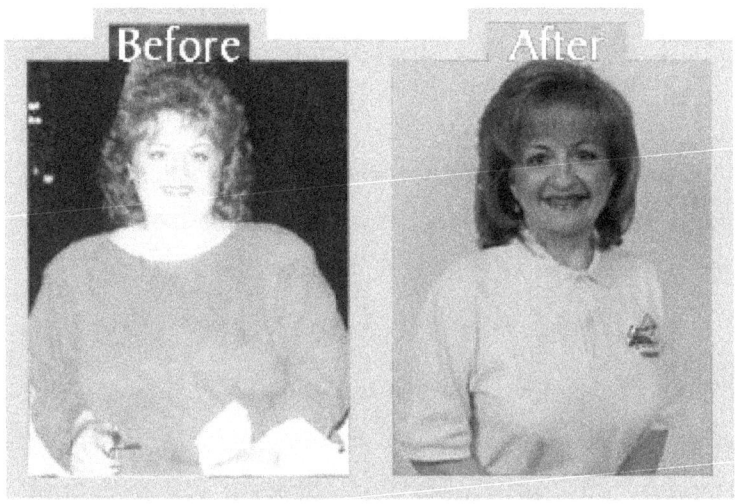

Since 1997, watching many clients with other trainers, and observing all my own clients over and over, the number one greatest thing about personal training is:

*AWESOME, ONE ON ONE, ACCOUNTABILITY!*

This is how it works: the majority of trainers work with clients two days a week for an hour each time. This is composed of a "one on one" meeting, by appointment. The appointment is always at the same time on the same two days. That is decided upon in the initial consultation.

Clients know, for instance, that at 10:00 a.m. on Tuesdays and Thursdays they will see their trainer and it quickly becomes a regular part of their lives. The trainer is waiting for you and you alone. Your hour has been paid for in advance and, therefore, you are more likely to show up! Also agreed upon initially is a "make-up" day in case the client has to re-schedule because of something that comes up, so there's no wriggling out of this. The trainer is there only and specifically for you, the client, at your chosen hour, and will devote THE ENTIRE TIME TO YOU!

*Because of the personal history I have in using so many well-known weight loss schemes, I understand how totally different this type of accountability is, and my reader with a similar history will immediately comprehend the significance of this difference.*

**The counselors I had in weight loss clinics did not even know if I had missed my meeting or not. They did not remember my name.** It is impossible for this to happen with personal training.

The trainer, at the initial consultation, may design a full cardiovascular and weightlifting program on paper for the client. This is based upon that client's goals and objectives, as well as any health and/or orthopedic issues. This meeting is normally free and the client walks away with this information, which is invaluable. Some trainers work **under the umbrella of a Registered Dietician**, and with an awesome software program they also design a nutrition regimen for their clients. This is like the food pyramid, a wide variety of foods, using your favorite foods, and a liberal, healthy number of calories. (The food pyramid is now choosemyplate.gov) It is a shame when clients trust a trainer on diet recommendations and the trainer is not under this umbrella.

*The individual program is very, very important because "one size does not fit all." It is extremely important for the client to start at a lowest point, which is, metabolically,* **results-oriented***, since he has often been* **doing nothing** *for a long time. This way the client has "somewhere to go," that is,* **progression which can be manipulated** *as his body becomes fitter and fitter. This also helps to overcome the dreaded "plateau" which causes so many clients to quit.*

Working on their own (or with a trainer on the TV weight loss challenge shows!) many times a client **starts** with the highest, most intense amount of exercise because they are in a hurry to get there. This never results in a lifetime permanent change. Many times this causes injury or emotional burnout. Also, leaving room to manipulate with **progression** in exercise helps the body with the dreaded plateau that comes up naturally after a certain amount of weight is lost. *A real plateau is when the food is right, the aerobic is right, the lifting is right, and still the scale does not move for a long time.* During this time you must have a trick to pull out of the bag to alter the metabolism. Where is the trick if you started with the highest amount when you did **not even need to start there to get results?**

It is during your weekly meetings with the trainer that you do an awesome weight lifting hour that is usually peppered with a great variety of exercises. This can vary with trainers as some nowadays will only teach "functional training" and use very little gym equipment.

During your weekly meetings with the trainer, she/he will ask you about your cardio/aerobic and nutrition *compliance*. They will help you with any problems you might encounter on that. They will manipulate your program with you as needed for progressions. Also, they will religiously measure you and weigh every 21 days (that is at least the Apex guide.) You must be honest with your trainer about how well you are adhering to the program, because the measurement every 21 days will reveal that anyway!

Many trainers I am familiar with don't weigh or measure more often than that because we teach the client to focus on the program and not on the scale. When we measure you, tape measures and body fat and changes in clothes sizes take *precedent* over what the scale says. The body fat analysis is very important. I use the three-pinch test that many Registered Dieticians teach. Women are pinched with a caliper in three different places and men are pinched with a caliper in three different places. A physics chart is used to determine body fat. It is best to always use the same trainer for this pinch test. It is a tool to show differences from one period to the next, and while it is somewhat subjective and not a pure science, it is a very good tool for both trainer and client that takes some of the focus off the scale. It becomes a very good tool as you stay with your trainer.

However, *when the Body Mass Index is high*, the scale must eventually come down also. I find that clients who are reading about weight lifting programs and gaining muscle mass will often use that new knowledge for a type of "denial" about the scale. If the BMI chart is very high, we must face the fact that even if we gain muscle, we must lose a lot of fat, and the scale comes down also dramatically eventually.

It is not the **same** as a person 5 - 10 pounds overweight who can actually lose inches and body fat from weight lifting and some cardio work while the scale remains the same. We must face facts about how overweight we really are. It is very difficult for some to face this.

It is **true** that when we lose weight the right way, (eating well with enough calories and exercising) that you can end up smaller in circumference at a much higher scale weight than in the past when you starved and did not exercise! But not 40 pounds over BMI!! That is denial!

While you are personally accountable for your program, your compliance and results are often based on personal lifestyle and other related issues that you must face. When I got Bariatric patients they were always about 5 years post op and starting to regain their weight. They had some food restrictions based on the surgery, but STILL needed accountability! Gaining weight back when you have had a successful surgery is very depressing and shocking. They need encouragement just as anyone does!

During the weekly meetings with my clients we will usually spend the first ten minutes going over their week together, to gauge how they are doing. Often they will come in and *before* I even ask them anything they brag how they have completed their aerobic program and recorded food records accurately and consistently. Sometimes, however, they complain to me that one area is weak, so we sit down and try to work on that weak area. Perhaps it is a time issue with exercise or maybe they finally recognize the need to get the boxes of ice cream out of the house and simply learn to enjoy the occasional scoop at Baskin Robbins. (**Surgery patients are often able to eat sweets. I can have sweets as long as they are heavily laid down with fat! No dumping! I can't eat sweets like sweet tea, jelly beans, icing on cake, fat free sweets, fat free ice cream, etc. Instead, I can eat the most fattening sweets!**) They may later be successful at going out and getting just one one scoop of ice cream like I do occasionally, but **not** keeping any in the house (**a skill power**) and still enjoying total satisfaction. However, they have discovered on their own that will power will not work with a ½ gallon of ice cream in the freezer. They are accountable for recognizing where they are weak, and in the final analysis, they are responsible for getting the ice cream out of the house.

As we weight lift for the next fifty minutes of their hour, we are also able to talk, but the client is aware that this is his own personal time for taking care of himself and he knows we have to use that session to work. The sessions are pre-paid (for example, the first twelve sessions are paid for upfront, and the next twelve are partially paid). And so, the sessions must be used to the advantage of the client. I never had accountability using any other program, and it was never personal. I did not feel my counselor was really my friend and was honestly concerned about me. Most of the time, he did not remember my name on sight. No one called me if I didn't show up. Perhaps two months down the road, someone from the company would call and ask where I had been. By then, I was too far gone, too deep in failure to start over.

**A Trainer's Job** (A quote from my American Council on Exercise study manual):

*In addition to providing ongoing expert advice and instruction about effective training for a client, a major part of the personal trainer's job is motivating the client to stick with a regular physical activity routine. Motivation, like other aspects of exercise, is a personal issue; what works for one client may not be successful for another. Developing strategies to keep each client interested and motivated will often be as important as designing the exercise program.*[16]

Susan, a recent client, was "ready" emotionally and spiritually. She had one trainer the previous year for six months and strictly complied with all the trainer told her. This was a trainer, about forty- five years old, from the "old school." There was no nutrition meeting. The trainer had always had a genetically gifted body and had always been a perfect eater, mainly focusing on the health food industry and relying on a variety of supplements. She never had to do a lot of cardiovascular activity herself and loved heavy weight lifting. **She was even a nurse, but she was teaching what had worked for <u>her all her life</u>**. Susan got zero results with this trainer. A trainer needs continual education in studying the <u>science</u> of the <u>different</u> goals/objectives of clients!

---

[16] Manual of the American Council on Exercise, Copyright 1996-97 Published by the American Council on Exercise

I had no openings when Susan first approached me, but I wanted to help her. On my calendar there would be an opening in a month so I told her to wait, but in the meantime to "get started" on her own. I advised her to join Weight Watchers because they are under the guidelines of Registered Dieticians and also teach an easy system to learn food values. Most importantly, they don't teach fast weight loss and they don't promote magic foods or bad foods. I told her to "work up" to walking three hours weekly and we discussed target zones she could work on. Susan had no health or orthopedic problems. She was only thirty-eight years old.

Well, once again Susan complied with instructions. By the time I got her for weight training a month later, she had already dropped ten pounds and was much fitter. Susan thought the previous year that having *any* trainer was "magic" and *strictly obeyed* the wrong instructions. Susan dropped sixty-five pounds in nine months! This was 15 months ago. She's back to a size eight and has not damaged her health or metabolism in the process. Now, for over a whole year, she has learned the science of "weight maintenance", something that she had never really absorbed.

A trainer can recognize if you are only doing the program to get into a wedding dress in three months. Most of them will talk you into a realistic goal that will not involve fast weight loss. I have turned down many a client after I saw they were only after fast weight loss.

Personal Trainers work hard for a living and we put much time, effort and *expense* into keeping our certification current and studying the science for each goal/objective and health issue. This is very, very individual. Make sure you are really hiring a Personal Trainer and not a fitness buff or a group instructor acting as a trainer. You want the *full benefit* of the standards we are held to in this business.

**The Personal Training business is still not held to many regulations or requiring a License. But there are many, many trainers who give themselves very good education, as I did. It is available to us. If I hired a trainer I would hire one with a current certification in ACSM, NASM, or ACE. However, the large organization that <u>accredits</u> certifications (NCAA) uses the <u>same criteria to approve all of them</u>.**

## Gym Science verses Real Science (Apex quote)

Most trainers nowadays take great pride in dispelling myths. They pound the truth into the client and subsequently, the client benefits. No matter how handsome or rich or well educated your fast weight loss MD is, he cannot alter the truth about how our metabolism works, or the effects of fast weight loss on our bodies.

**Following are just a few myths that a really good trainer will debunk. These myths are taken from Apex highly degreed kinesiology and nutrition experts. I stand on my "own life of denial and failures" in seeing their truths.**

**Myth:** "We can spot reduce certain areas of our bodies in the weight lifting room." False!

No such thing will happen. We can reduce fat all over our bodies with a whole body cardio workout and the right calories. We simply don't know where it will come off first or how much will come off where! Much of that is up to your genetic body build. Many responsible trainers feel betrayed by others who, by selling a product on TV, have convinced the public a certain product or piece of equipment can spot reduce.

**Myth:** "We get fat from too many carbs." False! We get fat from too many calories.

**Myth:** "We get fat from too much protein." False! We get fat from too many calories.

**Myth:** "We get fat from too much fat." False! We get fat from too many calories.

ENERGY UNITS IN – ENERGY UNITS OUT

**Myth:** "Eating after 6:00 p.m. makes us fat." False!

Too many calories consumed over a 24-hour period make us fat. (Although there is a consensus among Registered Dieticians that it is best to stop eating two hours before bedtime.)

**Myth:** "We can get thin from building lean body mass alone in the weight room." False!

The weight room helps to raise basal metabolism as muscle fiber grows. It is faster and more efficient to make sure you are doing enough cardiovascular activity to burn a lot of calories in order to be encouraged to continue. In aerobic activity the large muscles are working and the heart is sending a continuous supply of oxygen to keep up with these large muscles. Fat calories burn in the high, continuous presence of oxygen. Weight lifting is "start and stop." It is an anaerobic activity. Over the long haul, weight lifting will help you maintain your weight because after six months to a year, you will have more muscle! Five extra pounds of muscle burns 250 extra calories. That may not seem like much, but it helps you *to maintain once you have added calories back into your diet! Please note, that most females will not gain so much muscle that they will have an extraordinary new calorie burn. They will gain enough to help them maintain weight but it is not as much as males who have that testosterone hormone.*

**Myth:** "Only thin, fit people work out at athletic clubs." False!

I have worked in all types of gyms. There are many people who have serious weight problems attending the gym; I always see them being fully embraced, loved, and encouraged by everyone. The general public is impressed when an overweight person is obviously trying to make a change. You would receive continual validation from club members!

**Myth:** You can reach your weight loss goals with exercise alone, and eat about the same as you have been eating. False!

I have never seen someone start exercising, fail to change their calorie count by a few hundred, and still reach their weight loss goal. This is one of the values of food records. For example, based on the result of your own formula: Find out for sure if you have been gaining or maintaining on an average of 2,000 calories a day. Start an exercise program that won't burn you out and you will be able to keep it up. Then, make sure you are also deducting 500 calories a day from what you had been eating pre-exercise. Know your numbers = know your enemy.

*In order to maintain your new weight you can slowly add back in the 500 calories you took out as long as you continue to exercise. If I wanted to lose ten pounds, I know without a doubt that I would have to eat only 1,200 calories a day, while still exercising, instead of the 1500 that I maintain my weight on. Do your formula in Chapter Three!*

### "Prices"

In all clubs and with all trainers, the price per hour goes down dramatically if you buy a large package. Another good reason to purchase a large package is to learn as much as possible with the trainer at the very beginning, so you can become totally grounded over a period of time in all your new habits. I seldom sell anything but a three-month package. I truly believe I can have the most effect on a client if he is with me for an extended stretch while he makes adjustments in his lifestyle. When a client is with me for three months it is usually long enough for him to encounter a difficult "spell" with lifestyle issues, schedules, plateaus, and so forth. He will have professional support at a time when he might be tempted to quit and will remember those lessons when the going gets tough again, and he no longer has a trainer to help him through it.

In 2005, on the West Coast where I lived after the Hurricane, the large fitness club where I worked sold 18 one-hour sessions for $1,000. Many people bought these packages, at $55 a session. Today, in 2008, the largest athletic club here in the **South** where I live sells a 20-session one hour package for $800. This comes out to $40 a session.

Both of the above quotes are from large athletic clubs where the corporate structure is responsible for setting prices for personal training.

A trainer working from home does not have to pay a cut to the owners of the club. This is worth checking out, but be sure to SEE their certification history. And after years with many educational units their insurance will keep them on if the cert lapses.

There are also more affordable "very small group" sessions where 2-4 people share in the cost. The accountability in these small groups is also very good. There is normally an extra fee attached, but it brings down your hourly investment by $5-$10 per hour. You still get the same results and the same accountability, and for those who enjoy the company, it might even be more fun.

2020 UPDATE!! There are some great "online trainers" and they can hold you accountable. Prices are great!

You may want to check with self-employed trainers in small 24 hour fitness clubs. You may get a better price there. The trainers **appear t**o be employed as Staff members, but they are not. They simply pay the owners a cut of whatever they get and it is a win-win for the owners!

## How to find the right trainer

Whether you find a trainer from your large athletic club, a small club, a poster, or the Internet:

- Get his references and CALL them! Ask former clients about the results they are getting, most especially about accountability, promptness, and so forth.

- Read his entire resume and call some of the other non-client references.

- Do not take nutritional guidelines in detail from a trainer unless he is certified in nutrition under the umbrella of Registered Dieticians. If you like the trainer, and he is not certified in nutrition, go to Weight Watchers *simultaneously* while training with him.

- Make sure you see his certification history. If he is affiliated with a club, the club's staff will have his papers on file and they have approved his certification history.

- Of course, a trainer who has been certified for years has taken countless educational units and that is *definitely* in your favor. A trainer who has worked at a large athletic club has worked with many clients and has been in alliance with physical therapists. This is also in your favor.

- Even if you seem to have a great rapport with a young or recently certified trainer, make sure he has a mentor. The mentors are great! New trainers are so excited about doing a good job that they are simultaneously absorbing energy and motivation from both their mentors and their clients! You will benefit from the relationship with a mentor, and most especially from the trainer's fresh excitement.

- Make sure your trainer is insured if he is not affiliated with a club. Otherwise, the club has made certain he is insured.

- If he doesn't do a health consultation and doesn't talk to you about what you should "avoid" because of your bad knee, bad elbow, etc., this is a definite Red Flag! Most qualified trainers will address this in the initial consultation. But, you must tune into your own body and be truthful with your trainer. Trainers are not "mind reading genies," though we often read between the lines from seeing the same thing over and over!

- If you have a serious health or orthopedic issue, and he doesn't ask for a physician's release, this is another Red Flag. The release is normally sent to your physician, with a written program description attached, asking for areas where the physician wants limitations.

- Work with the trainer free-of-charge for one whole hour and make certain you feel comfortable with each other's personalities. This is important. You will be spending a lot of time with this person and the relationship can affect your progress.

Working with the trainer for a free hour will also let you know if you enjoy his style in the weight room. One overweight, middle- aged lady already working with a trainer came to me in desperation and said, "Please let me hire you! I came to this guy simply to get off the couch, learn a good exercise program and lose body fat; not spend all my time balancing on one leg!" It was a funny comment that I will not soon forget. By the same token, some clients would prefer that trainer's program to my own. It all depends on what you are looking for, so the initial try-out session before you pay up can save you a lot of frustration in the long run. There are now many wonderful training "techniques" on the floor with a trainer who is not a "dinosaur" in the industry! I use a great variety, and do not focus on just one technique (circuit training, negative training, isolateral training, functional training, balance training, free weights, cable equipment, slow training, the list goes on and on so you will never get bored!) The investment in a trainer for at least three months may cause you to think of weight lifting as a "hobby and play", rather than "working out". That is priceless.

Get the *best accountability* in the world with the right trainer for you. The right trainer will listen to you and design a program for you based upon your goals, your health issues, your injuries, and all your hang-ups.

**EMBRACE A Lifetime Program!**

# CHAPTER SEVEN

## *FIND A "PAM'S BULLET" THAT MAY BE LIFE CHANGING.*

If people like us could just go to a less "developed" country for one year and have our metabolism and minds changed by a forced regular diet of healthy, natural foods in normal portions accompanied by many hours of walking and hard physical work each week, we might realize that our American lifestyle is at the heart of the obesity epidemic. However we live in the United States and short of joining the Peace Corps we will continue to be confronted by volumes of rich food whenever we leave the house We will continue to feel that we "don't have time" to exercise because of "hurried" lifestyle here in America!

### From the Mayo Clinic:

*Within the first two years following surgery, you can expect to lose 50% to 60% of your excess weight, if you follow the dietary and exercise recommendations. If you continue to follow these recommendations, you can keep off most of this weight long-term. However, if you return to your old eating habits, you may gain back any weight you've lost. People who regain weight after gastric bypass surgery usually are consuming too many high calorie foods and beverages and don't exercise enough. And rather than eating three meals a day and small snacks, some people **graze** and eat food all day* long. This eating pattern often leads to consuming too many calories, which causes weight gain.[17]

## Food Bullet Tips to Consider

- *Planned Cheating*: So much of binging, purging, bulimia, and other eating disorders have much to do with guilt and self-punishment...the attitude of, "I don't dare to eat a chocolate bar. I don't deserve to eat a chocolate bar. I'm a bad person and a failure if I eat a chocolate bar. I hate myself so why not eat a chocolate bar and prove how unlovable I am!" This does not exist when I allow myself to eat a chocolate bar as part of my plan because it isn't something horrible and I control whether I eat it or not; it doesn't control me! I think psychologically one of the most important changes I made in my life was when I stopped punishment/reward eating. Whenever I choose to eat a chocolate bar or any other high- calorie sweet, I simply re-adjust my calorie bound*aries* with a very low-calorie, balanced meal, full of fiber and flavor, to create fullness and satisfaction. I experience no guilt simply because I ate a chocolate bar; rather, I enjoy it as it was meant to be enjoyed!

    A key to my weight control was not to be hungry,

---

[17] MAYO CLINIC. Com. October 4, 2005 GASTRIC BY-PASS SURGERY PAGE 3 OF 3 Weight Loss and Weight Regain. This is a warning from the surgeons themselves about your capacity to eat too much.

while staying in my calorie boundaries. This was by eating and exercising in a balanced way.

- Instead of looking only at a single day of food records, I looked at a **"seven-day average."** The seven-day average always made me feel in my mind that I had done well and achieved a "balanced diet" over the week. All my clients have reported having the same experience. For example: I maintain my weight now on 1,500 calories a day, a wide variety of healthy foods and some small treats. Seven days times 1,500 equals 10, 500 a week. I only estimate the calories (it works with your exercise program as your "ace in the hole.") I add the calorie estimate for seven days and it could come to 11,300. Hey, I thought I did badly! But I was only 800 calories over for the entire week. I could still maintain on that. Using a 7 day average helped me not to feel like I had axe-murdered my mother over just one day that was not in line with my daily calorie allowance! We lose the battle when we feel guilty!

- Adopt a vision of a healthy weight. Say it out loud daily and if it fits into God's principles in the Word, there is no reason you cannot have this vision. By the way, a healthy weight does fit into God's principles for many biblical reasons. Some *people will be naturally a bit heavier and still healthy.* God designed our bodies to be healthy and that includes having a *healthy weight, which does not result in unnecessary health issues for you.* You are the one who must determine what your healthy weight is, considering health issues. A body fat analysis should be used in some cases also. There is more on this in Chapter Six. Be realistic and be satisfied with a higher weight as long as it is not so high that it can produce health issues.in other area of our lives! The higher your weight is the more calories you can have to maintain! Lifetime maintenance is the biggest victory!

- Walking and eating many small meals within your calorie/ carb/fat/and protein level, and having a healthy weight can cure and prevent Type II diabetes! (Type 1 diabetes is a different entity and is not caused by lifestyle.)

- I dropped the habit of weighing on the scale daily. That always sabotaged my mind because the scale often deceives with fluid weight, as many females are well aware! Instead, I only weighed weekly. I actively filled my mind with something positive before I weighed. I tried on formerly snug clothes *(clothes that used to be tight on me and were now loose told me more about my loss in inches than the scale did)* and took tape measurements so that I could see progress and not just depend on the scale. I replaced the mental fear of the scale with practical habits which worked to encourage me no matter what the scale said that day. I now only weigh myself about six times a year, and depend on the fit of my clothes and tape measurements to let me know where I stand at any given moment. I also check body fat analysis twice a year. *You must have the courage to try on your snuggest clothes each week.* As you get closer to your goal weight, the weight loss will become slower. People just can't seem to embrace this. We continue to be impatient and the evil one uses this impatience to destroy our final goal.

**Remember "God's timing is perfect"**

- More about the scale: "Picture this" – a spoiled <u>one pound</u> package of hamburger meat! That is what only a <u>one pound</u> weight loss looks like on a smaller body! When we are very overweight, it takes many pounds to really see a smaller body! But, when we are closer to the goal weight, although the weight goes down much slower, the offset of that is that even one pound shows a lot! Say this positive truth to yourself when the weight loss is slow! Talk back to your demons with an attitude! I talk back to them with scripture. Jesus says in Matthew that man does not live on bread alone, but on the very word of God! Even Jesus had to use scripture when fighting Satan!

    *Claim* **First Peter 5:8** *"Be self-controlled and alert, for the evil one is prowling around looking for a victim to devour. Resist him, and in a short while, God will lift you up to high ground!"*

***1 John 4:4!*** *"He that is inside of us is greater than He who is in the world."*

***1 Corinthians 10:13.*** *"God will give us a way of escape in temptation."*

- I identified foods which made me "feel good" within twenty minutes of eating them. Surgery patients are forced to do this, but actually all people should do it. As we identify these foods, we will prefer the choice that makes us feel really good for a few hours, that is, light and full of energy rather than sluggish and heavy. For instance, a grilled cheese sandwich with a sliced tomato on it makes me feel great for hours, so I have that for breakfast most mornings. A bowl of cereal, even a low-sugar brand with low-fat milk, leaves me feeling less energetic only 30 minutes after eating.

- I identified foods which "filled me." These were low-calorie, high-fiber veggies. I kept bowls of cut cucumbers on hand daily, marinated in low calorie "Wish Bone" Italian dressing (16 calories). I sometimes added sliced onions to them for a little variety. I had at least two delicious tomatoes every day on which I smeared my favorite diet mayo. I had low fat popcorn at night in a "mini-bag" and the fiber made me feel very satisfied before bed time. Staying full was important to keep Satan's tricks at bay.

- I identified foods which gave me my "sweet fix." Low calorie popsicles (15 calories each) gave me the sweet fix I needed while I was on 1,200 calories. I could have built a castle with those sticks! The cold popsicles also took a long time to finish which satisfied my psychological oral need for food, rather than a true feeling of hunger. Fat free fudge sticks gave me a real "cheat." Once, I ate the whole box while very upset. However, I am glad that they were there as the six fudge sticks only came to 300 calories and I was still within calorie boundaries for that day. Now, years later, I just make sure I have "part of something sweet" and work it into my calories for the day. I re-adjust with some delicious veggies for my last meal and stay full. Other people may not understand how we are, but we have to fight "fire with Fire" until we get better. I got better over time, but the tricks were essential and I still use all my tricks as and when needed. "Know thine enemy!"

- I worked hard to anchor a new habit of religiously keeping my house food-proofed (or food friendly) in essence, keeping my favorite healthy foods and snacks always available while keeping unhealthy foods that I was sure to devour in a moment of stress or fatigue out of the house. When this new habit had really been anchored in my mind and life for a long time, I found myself automatically not using the wrong foods at home, even when they were present for some reason. But the new habit had to be securely anchored first. Please notice that this is an example of "skill power, not will power, as discussed in a previous chapter.

- I got into the habit of putting my "body" on my calendar, not just my never-ending to-do list. My body was there on my Day-Timer with directions to "walk, and record food records."

- I had always gone by a to-do list and Day-Timer. Putting my body on the calendar as a priority helped me to keep my commitment on my mind; I couldn't avoid it, it was visibly present on my to-do list! Anchoring this new habit of including myself on the list eventually helped me to stop saying "I don't have time" because I always get my list done! When my body became part of the list, it stopped being expendable.

- I kept daily food records and educated myself with a lifetime nutrition program. It takes five minutes a day and you can eventually learn to estimate, so that you don't have to look it up in a book forever. (See Resource Page)

- Focus on "simpler" meals and foods which are much easier to estimate on calorie boundaries. For example, a deliciously seasoned small chicken breast (3-4 ounces – the size of a woman palm of her hand) instead of a chicken casserole. Serve the rice (size of a woman's fist) on the side. You will learn that the chicken breast is 35 calories per ounce as long as it is skinned. You will learn that the rice is about 100 calories for that portion. It is an estimate, but you will come much closer to right estimates with simpler eating.

- For complex foods, for your estimate, I have found that my estimates are very close to correct, and much less stressful, by doing the following: I eat some delicious frozen meals or canned meals. I have some favorites. I like the Healthy Choice soups and the Healthy Choice frozen meals most of all. When I eat them, I notice the portion sizes and the calories listed on the can or package. I just save these packages and can labels. When I eat some complex meals at home or at a restaurant, I just estimate by copying the calorie/fat gram levels from these complex foods. For example, a whole can of Healthy Choice Soup, for the chili soup, was 325 calories. For the same amount of my own homemade chili, using the lean meat, I would use the same calorie and the same can amount. For my own homemade spaghetti, I would use the frozen meal and the calorie amounts. This was an effort at first, but now it is very easy. When at a restaurant, I use the same concept, but from the canned or packaged frozen meals that are not advertised as low calorie or low fat. I always fill up on green salads or low calorie veggies first, with low calorie dressings.

- Mentally, I reminded myself out loud on a daily basis to focus on the journey, not the destination, and to forsake fast weight loss. With time, I *actually embraced* slower weight loss. Waiting on God's perfect methods is very difficult, but I said out loud daily, "Focus on your food program and discoveries, focus on your walking," and I waited on God's promise to reward my patience.

- I made a great discovery of eating an early lunch or dinner if I was hungry. Eating a balanced meal earlier than usual, instead of waiting until I was starving, was one of the best changes I made. Now, many years later, if I am tempted to eat too much of something rich, I use my skill power and instead eat a balanced, tasty meal on the spot to satisfy my natural hunger.

- Maintenance is a victory! If you are not losing, but just maintaining your weight, turn that fact into a positive force in your mind. If you have been steadily gaining weight for years, and are only maintaining your present weight, say to yourself "maintenance is a victory." Perhaps you are on a long plateau which is explained in Chapter Three. Perhaps life has truly just been so tough lately, that you need to say to yourself, "I am not going to challenge myself for the next two weeks with a weight loss amount of calories, but I am going to take myself "off the hook", and just work at MAINTENANCE! This awful lifestyle challenge which I am now in (perhaps a death or a job change, etc.) will be over soon and I will be back to developing a good, new normal routine. Then I will go back to the weight loss challenge, but halleluiah, I will not begin from that "pit of having gained weight back!"

**"I will begin again from maintenance, which has required some effort also!"**

- Most of all, stop believing promotional campaigns and listening to offbeat stuff. There are no magic foods, there are no bad foods. There are percentages. Richer foods are to be eaten in smaller portions. The calorie is the bottom line. It is an Energy Unit.... A Fuel unit... beautiful word!

**Exercise Bullets:**

- It is very important to re-discover "play" in the area of regular exercise. If it continues to be just an obligation for you, you will eventually give up.

- Use music or a book tape instead of depending on a partner. If you do it inside, enjoy a TV show you would watch anyway.

- Put your exercise time on your "day timer" each and every time that you make out your "to do" list.

- When you absolutely have to skip a week or two for some good reason, say out loud and believe to yourself, "starting over is awesome!"

- It is important that you examine "time efficiency" for your exercise program. For example: is it really necessary to go all the way to the gym when you could do your cardio right outside your door or in front of your TV? If we make these

- 2.5 or 4 hours per week of cardio exercise fit into our schedules, and then we will be more likely to keep doing it. I enjoy my cardio right outside my door or at my Marina when I am boating anyway. I keep a bike and a kayak there and walk the piers with a wonderful view.

- When should you exercise? There are many scientific studies on "when" is the best time to get the most out of your exercise. The answer from my perspective using my history and watching my clients is the best time is the easiest available time that you have in your busy schedule, because you WILL DO IT! The difference between not doing the exercise time and actually doing it is the biggest difference of all. For two years, I did it at night consistently… only time that I could. For two years I did it at lunch time consistently because it was the only time I had. For five years I did it at 5:00 in the morning! For four years, I have mostly used midday or afternoon. Now I am back to morning. It has to be on my schedule. It is SCHEDULED!

**Choose the time when you will be consistent and frequent. That works!**

- If you continue to view a regular exercise program only as a means for weight loss, rather than for weight maintenance, you probably won't be successful over time.

- If you adopt an unbalanced view of exercise with regards to "how much, how intense, and how often," you will not experience "joy or return to play;" you will probably encounter burnout or injury.

- Do not buy into myths such as "spot reducing," or thinking you have to be a "runner" rather than a walker. You will be frustrated when you discover that 500 crunches a day have not made your stomach flat. You will be disappointed and frustrated when you become injured running, when you are not a runner (this is very common) and then you can't do anything at all!

- Adopt an attitude of CONSISTENCY, FREQUENCY, and MODERATION. Moderation is the key as it will lead to LIFETIME consistency and frequency, making exercise a regular part of your life, not something you constantly quit and restart, over and over. My mom is seventy-nine and still takes long, long power walks (up hills a lot) and does a challenging Pilates class. She has never over done it...... and she has never stopped. She has never been overweight. She has never been on a diet. She has always eaten everything, including treats, in moderation.

- Believe that "calories in and calories out" is the only magic formula out there. Energy intake, energy expenditure. Take calories in and burn them up. Extra calories left in the body, according to your **own personal physics** formula in Chapter Three, will be stored as fat.

- If you continue to believe that "one size fits all", that little Suzie Body Builder next door has the routine that will make you look like her, that there are magic workouts, magic machines, or magic personal trainers, you will be frustrated. Why? Because it isn't true! An exercise program must be designed specifically for WHERE YOU ARE at a given time, and it should follow and progress to where you go over time. The exercise program must change as you change, and progress as you progress, but the "magic" is in doing the exercise that is right for you at that time.

- Do not insist that all your mundane, daily household chores (yes, I do them too!) and responsibilities must be completed before your forty minutes of scheduled exercise time. Those never-ending tasks will deplete your energy. Trust me: your mundane chores will be less mundane if you do the forty minutes first!

**I still say to myself out loud, "I will put this time first, God. I will trust that I am able to complete my other chores and my other errands later that are weighing on my mind. I know that the evil one will steal this exercise time from me if I put every single chore and errand in front of it."**

- Once you identify and recognize the increased energy and enhanced mood level that regular, aerobic exercise provides, you will look forward to it with excitement; it will no longer be an obligation.

- Many times we make the mistake of only exercising if we are also doing well following a balanced food program. But, if we "fail," that is, if we fall off the food program (not being perfect) we decide we are just failures through and through, become discouraged and negative and decide we might as well not exercise either. *Why keep trying if you have fallen from perfection?* This "demonic mentality" is common among people who are dealing with obesity. That was truly one of the most self-defeating mindsets that I experienced. I assure you that whenever you get away from your food program, whatever it is, if you stick with the exercise program you will continue to feel good about that at least, it will keep you from falling so low that you give up entirely, and it will *encourage you to get back on track with the food program again.*

- Do not get on the scale right away when you have been away from part of your program. Wait one week, after being on the nearly perfect program (food, cardio, and lifting). Many times we will show a great deal of "sodium" weight gain and because we have not been doing "perfect," then we become defeated if we think the relatively benign imperfections resulted in a 3-5 pound weight gain. Wait a week!

- Leave your messy exercise clothes and shoes out in a place where you have to "walk over them." That is your cue to pick them up and go. Leave your music (I-pod or whatever) on top of it. Don't clean this mess up!

- If hair is a problem because of sweat and it becomes straight as a board when you exercise, work on that problem. If lunchtime is a time you could really exercise and get it out of the way, then go to war and get a cute hairpiece for after lunch. God will do miracles for you if you are determined to exercise at the time that is really best for you. I exercised at work, at lunchtime, for two years. I worked it out!

- If your regular time to exercise changes, write up a note to yourself about your brand new plan and until this time and plan becomes automatic in your brain! Look at the note and say it out loud. It will become automatic soon.

## MORE HELP ON FINDING TIME

Unfortunately, we often seem to have the **"all-or-nothing"** mentality in this country with regard to exercise. If we can't be top fit and participate in every sport, if we can't run a five-mile marathon, if we can't leave the kids at home and go to the gym five days a week. If we can't DO IT ALL, then what do we do? NOTHING!

It simply isn't true that we don't have time to improve our fitness level; don't have time to exercise moderately; don't have time to play actively outdoors with our kids on the weekends. However, our tendency is to make a lot of excuses, and the main one is, "I don't have time to exercise." When we don't make that time, we soon get so out of shape (spending our "time" on the couch in front of the TV or glued to the computer screen) we can no longer enjoy doing these things.

So stop making excuses, and start looking for a comfortable midpoint between ALL and NOTHING that fits your lifestyle and schedule.

As you view the important following chart, do some brainstorming. Write your ideas down on this chart. What motivates you? Your spouse? Your kids? Paste their photos on the chart! Do you want to be able to take your kids jet-skiing on a river, but don't have the fitness level to do that safely? Put a picture of a Jet Ski on the chart. Is there a Bible verse or a saying that will inspire and motivate you to start exercising and stay with it? *I love mine: Isaiah 40:31: "They will soar on wings like eagles; they will run and not grow weary, they will walk and not be faint."* Write it down on the chart!

Then make some copies of your chart and hang them on your mirror, your fridge, your office desk, wherever you will see them frequently. Internalize these ideas and goals. "Hypnotize" yourself into thinking and believing that this is possible for you!!

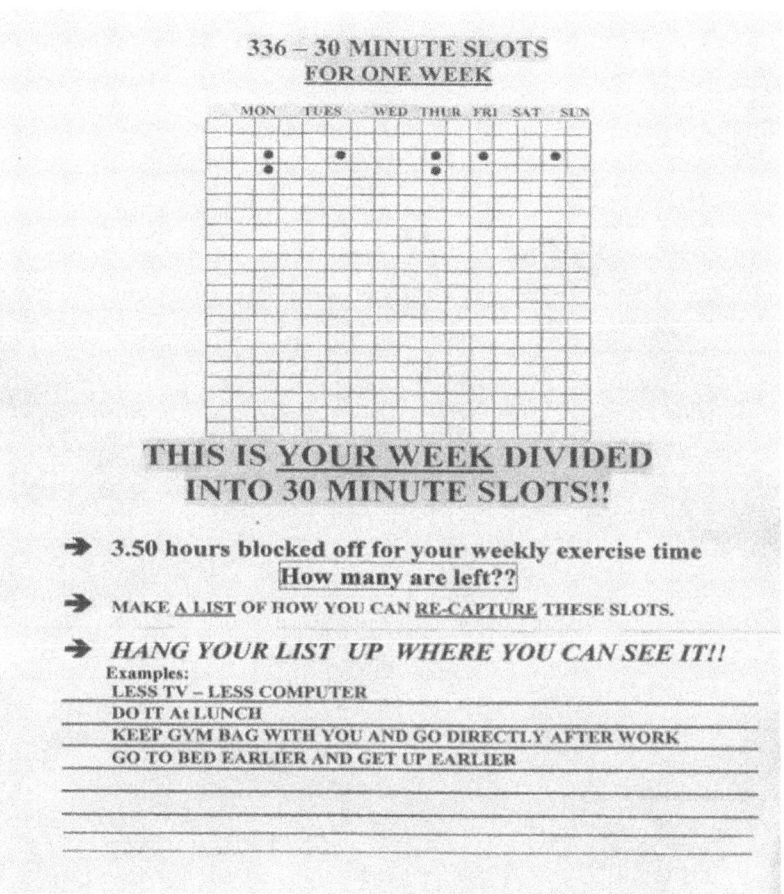

CHART FROM 1996 PUBLICATION OF NATIONAL STRENGTH AND CONDITIONING ASSOCIATION.

Al and I always said we had "no time." We wasted **our time saying we had no time!** If we had only discovered earlier that a mere 3 ½ hours a week of consistent, moderate exercise actually builds about ten more hours of energy and vitality into your week. Believe me, this is a small investment for a priceless return.

# CHAPTER EIGHT

## *IMPORTANT UPDATE ON PAM AT AGE 69 (THE BULK OF THIS MANUSCRIPT WAS WRITTEN AT AGE 58)*

I give most of the credit for a larger percentage of surgery patients **maintaining** most of their weight loss directly to those patients who have become **Internet bloggers.**

This massive correspondence of worldwide patients between each other has forced the clinics to be totally honest and *more* helpful. Therefore, the clinics now **must admit** that the surgery can be "outeaten" and "under exercised" after the *window of total ease has ended* (in most cases two – four years.) The clinics must now include exercise help and nutritional information to the patients. This is very apparent in all of the blogging sites where thousands of patients blog.

**Previous to this blogging there was little or no information from post op patients about their maintenance stories.** Patients just "disappeared," many of them "shamed into silence." I had no contact with anyone about my struggles in 1980 and in 1995. But later, I realized I was not alone as I got several post op Personal Training clients who were regaining their weight. Also, when Carnie Wilson came out in 2006 about her regain, I knew I was not alone.

I had felt horrified and alone for a long time with "my secret" that the bariatric surgery was not foolproof. It was *widely marketed and shouted on media* and among medical professionals that the anatomical changes were so severe that no one could possibly re-gain any weight. I was successful myself in a slow, complete weight loss, but I could comfortably eat way beyond my calorie requirements very early on and felt horrified and shocked based on what I was told and what was reality.

I thank God for the Internet bloggers. They are now a powerful force in Bariatric surgery, pre-op and post-op. My favorite blogging site is **"Bariatric Foodie."** Nikki manages the site well and is very balanced in her approach and in the academics of nutrition and exercise. She is also very prolific in the surgeries and in great vitamin recommendations which are so important for Bariatric surgery. She is also not *afraid* of the word Calorie!

However, her primary focus is on great nutrition, good vitamins, and recipes designed for patients. She leads the blogging well, especially for those who are very depressed about struggling again. I recommend reading this blog daily and contributing your own help to the patients from time to time. It will be mutual! It is far better than any psychiatric help that a food addicted patient can get, and it is FREE! Greater numbers are really set free now from food addiction, starting with surgical intervention. **However, the substantial number who regain after 5 to 10 years is very disturbing.**

**October 29, 2019:** I just watched **The Today Show** on NBC. Al Roker interviewed a recent Gastric By-pass patient. It was refreshing to hear them saying things like "this is not the end, it is only the **means** to the end", and we must change our mindset before the "honeymoon" ends." **Note from Pam:** in the 1990's the media only presented this as an outright miracle. In my opinion that hurt more than it helped and as a result of this approach a large majority gained all their weight back.

**Changes in my life at an older age. We finally do age!**

I am 69 years old now and 25 years post –op. I have five grandkids now, ages 16 down to 7. I am very active with them. Although life changes, I still feel young for my age. I still boat year round. I still kayak year round. I still bike year round with the wind and the sun in my face and it still makes me feel as if I am 30 years old… or a *child at play!!* I still lift weights, but lightly. I still do housework and yard work with a new house closer to the five grandkids who enjoy their very active Mi-Mi. My boat and kayak and one of my bikes are at a Marina close by, instead of in my backyard on a waterfront property.

I went back to a large, progressive athletic club in 2017 and work with a few personal training clients. I have one or two clients come to my home gym. This is to keep me busy now that the grandkids are older and branching out to friends and the world. I still feel retired and my life at home is first priority and the 6-8 hours a week of work is just fun, not stressful. I am there about the same amount of time that the other seniors are, but they are just socializing and working out!

**As to the changes that come with aging?** I no longer jog. I no longer jet ski. Pounding my back is not good. I no longer lift heavy weights in the gym. I miss racquet sports but dangerous for my spine.

Gastric By-pass **S**urgery is responsible for the full blown Osteoporosis that I have had since age 63. I have lost 2.5 inches in height. My spine x-ray looks like a Capital S instead of a nice straight spine. The bone loss affected what had been my "slight" Scoliosis. My thyroid has gone up and down where it had been stabilized for years previous to my surprising early 60's.

However, the rest of my blood profile and health looks "like a 30 year old's" as expressed by my General Practitioner. I would like to think that some of those good numbers are because I have spent 25 years in a new lifestyle! Some of it is certainly just good genetics!

If I am fortunate enough to become elderly I certainly realize that some of these numbers will worsen simply because of age. The body wears out and mine has already started! My only medicine right now is thyroid medicine and vitamins! I do not take bone density medicine but use other means to keep it stable. This is my *personal preference* after the study of bone density medications. My bone density has remained stable for the last four years.

Vitamins are better designed now to protect bariatric patients. In 1995 the vitamins were not as effective at protecting us. I was in denial that my plumbing was radically surgically changed and now different from that of a normal person. I have paid a big price for that.

Information has changed so much that I am a dinosaur regarding the surgeries in some regards, compared to current blogging sites. My book will, however, always be *timeless* I hope.

The flatuation is also worse and that is embarrassing. Of course we all know that it is seldom toxic, but very loud!!! For years it only occurred after bedtime. Now it can be a surprise after relaxing in the daytime, especially when just getting up from a sitting position. I have changed my diet just a little to reflect the bariatric pyramid more in order to *offset* the flatuation. For years I was able to comfortably eat more of a "choosemyplate.gov" diet and only avoid foods that caused dumping or fatigue.

I was a very spoiled patient! I had literally no problems or side effects for years until this recent aging process. I think that this very long period of excellent health made me complacent in protecting myself with the proper vitamins. **I felt like the bionic woman for decades**! I was extremely slender at 5 ft. tall, **and** athletic and healthy, with few side effects.

**FITNESS:** I am **only 4 ft. 9 and half inches** now! This is legally a "little person!" The chart in Chapter Three lists height as affecting our calorie burn, our BMR. It certainly has affected mine.

**My inability to exercise with great *intensity* has changed because I have to *protect my spine*. The lack of exercise intensity that I practiced for years, once I was a fitter person, has affected my calorie burn. (Intensity is required as a fit**

**person in order to maintain. Duration is required in the beginning as an unfit person.)**

The thyroid was way down for a whole year the first time and I did not catch it. It is now corrected and I keep a close eye on it. I refuse to diet and lower my calories from the comfortable 1500 that I have maintained on since post menopause at age 55. I am *maintaining the new weight*, which I will be happy about at this age. The pouch is still strong and I am satisfied with small meals and would never be able to binge…. praise God. Bingeing was my primary food addiction, which the surgery *on its very own* delivered me from forever. For me, bingeing required stealing, lying, and cheating. This increased my sadness in regard to my faith and obedience to my Lord.

As a result of all of these *old age changes*, I am two sizes larger but **still** fairly small! Thank God that I "went for the gold" in 1996 and became as small as I did! I have never fallen off the wagon…. Praise God!

*Maintenance is a Victory at Any Weight!*

To be honest, I must struggle emotionally from time to time with my shorter and thicker body at this older age because I was a "noted trainer" for decades who wrote books and gave motivational presentations. *It absolutely and totally humbles me.* However, as a believer and follower of Christ, I know that this humbling experience **renews** my compassion for the morbidly obese and all bariatric patients. After all these years I have *again remembered firsthand what the struggle was like for 38 years.*

However, I have once again also **taken my stand against falling prey** to rapid weight loss schemes and exercise inactivity. I have a **renewed stand** in regard to all the information in all of my chapters! **It is all true. We still have the truth! Just as I did in 1996, when I came to the "end of myself" in Chapter One, and decided to take action God's way, I still embrace that. The Rest of the Truth, the whole truth!**

I will also just be happier at this older age at a larger size but will do *all the work necessary* to maintain this new size for my health! I am a healthy and fit aged 69 grand-ma. I thank God for that *renewed* compassion for the feelings of the obese. I remember how my husband and I suffered with sadness, especially with the guilt that as a Christian we could do nothing about this but mutilate our bodies! I am at peace with that now and appreciate God's kind and permissive help!

I still feel that I can speak to these issues that affect food addiction, and perhaps better than ever even though I am no longer "the lean mean, young fighting machine" that I was!"

I have **never dropped the "holy habits" that God taught me and that I hope will help others.** .

I forgot **how** to be food addicted and **I still tell myself** "I can't wait to exercise tomorrow!" Adopting **moderation** instead of fast weight loss led to **consistency** and **frequency** in food and exercise for a **lifetime.**

**This can happen for you as well!** I am still amazed at how the Lord taught me one little step at a time, and *changed me totally* from the very food addicted and sedentary person that I was. **Success is incremental and comes in percentages….. God changed me one fraction at a time and <u>forever!</u>**

**1 Corinthians 3:18.** "The Lord **changes** us from little too little, from glory to glory." I guess I seem a little crazy to girlfriends at age 69 who ask me to do to sedentary type events. I am often far too busy on my boat or cleaning my boat on its boat slip, on my kayak, or on my bike! I live for this and those **active hobbies still set me on fire** after so many years of being "nailed to the ground!" Yesterday at 69 years of age the ladder broke on the boat as I attempted to go from kayak to boat off of the river. I was able to hang on for a long time until someone could rescue me! I am still agile and active for someone my age, but **ver**y cautious so that I can remain active and not be incapacitated with my spine.

I still long to help those *younger* people to change their lives in order to *run and play* with their kids and grandkids. I know that they want to be an example of Godly health and fitness to the generations below them that they love so much. I know that they want to protect them from the same problems they have had in this area. I still long to help those *middle aged* people to avoid an early death as in my husband's case. And I hope this **update** encourages *older* people to keep their holy habits because we need them now *more than ever!*

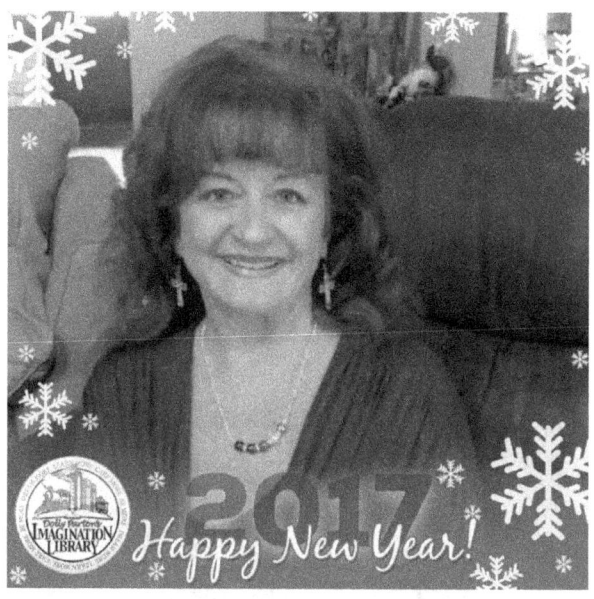

*A good close-up in 2017. My grandchildren's birthstones on a necklace they gave me!*

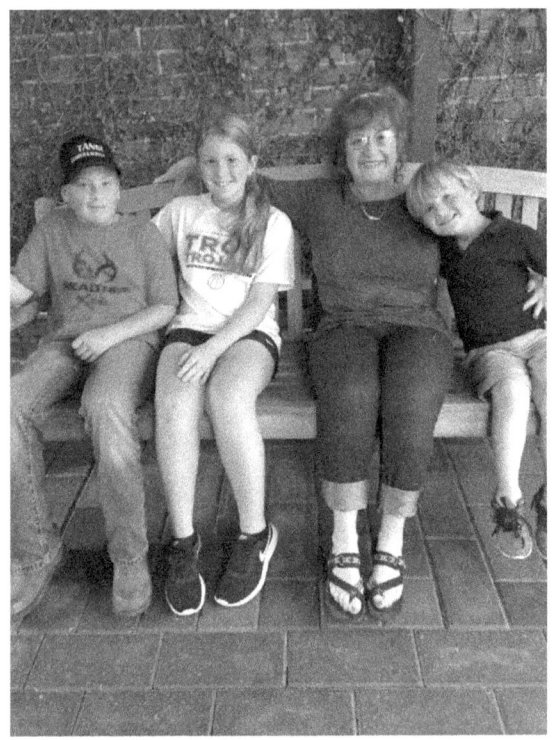

*2017. My Feet are not touching the floor at my new height! Toes are pointed!*

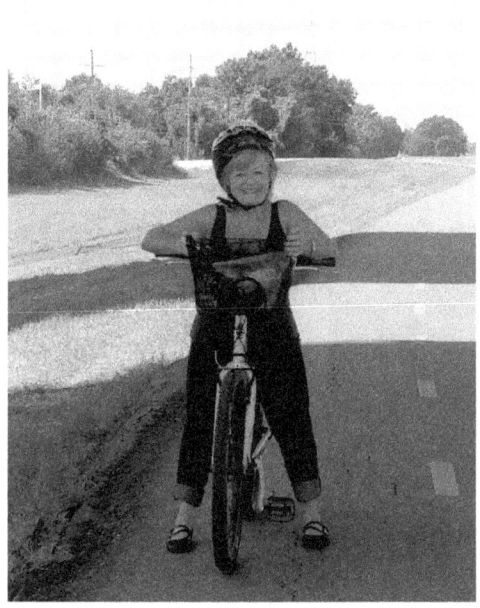

*I can hardly see over the handle bars now at this shorter height! I almost fall off trying to get my leg over the bike! If you look, no waistline anymore!*

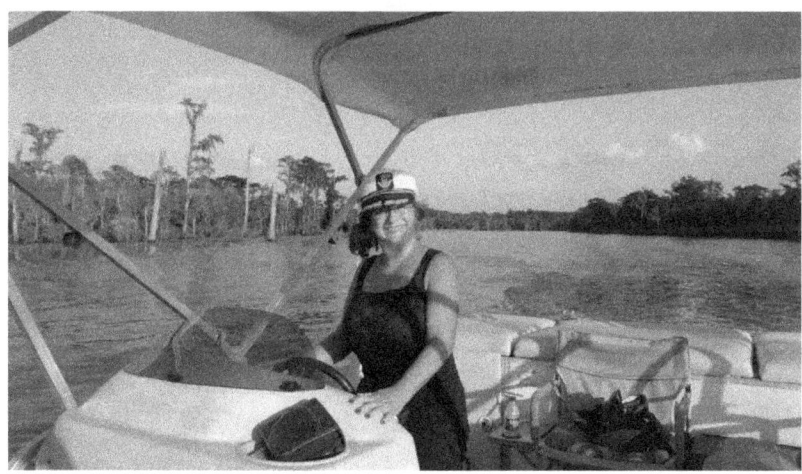

*Little thicker, age 68.... Still a sassy boat captain. I keep kayaks on the boat and throw them out in different places on the River. In 1996 I promised God no more sedentary hobbies. At least hobbies that move some or require activity in setting up. I had to get a kayak that did not hurt my back. I call the boat my boyfriend! He is!*

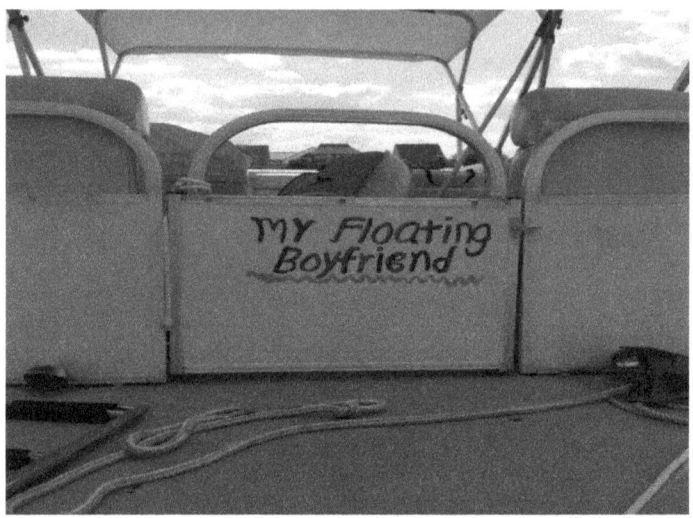

*He only requires a little rub down at times! I am the boss! LOL*

# CHAPTER NINE

## *REDEEMED BY GOD'S GRACE. LET GOD WRITE HIS STORY INTO OURS!*

I was baptized 47 years ago at age 22. Three months earlier I had experienced a "Damascus Road" conversion. The alternative to that conversion was death, or prison, or more mental hospitals. I came from a very good home and we were in church, as was politically correct in the 50's and 60's. My family practiced great Christian principles. But vocally they were raised to be very private about their faith and prayer, even at home. This is very common. I ended up being agnostic. My family in the last two decades has changed to quite "warm and fuzzy and even vocal about their faith," and has remained very faithful to Christ and the church. I am so very grateful that in elementary school we were required to go to church. That was pivotal in my conversion later! God's word does not return void and it will accomplish what it sets out to do.

**Isaiah 55:11 King James Version (KJV)** So shall my word be that goeth forth out of my mouth: it shall not return unto me void, but it shall accomplish that which I please, and it shall prosper in the thing whereto I sent it.

In hindsight and with all that has been researched and summarized in the mental health industry during the last decade, I believe that something happened to my brain at birth in a <u>severe breech</u> (buttocks first) delivery where mothers die sometimes and babies have brain injury. We each survived that surprisingly well, it appeared. In my opinion, *as my brain grew* past young childhood, social sharpness and proper development lagged behind. My parent's first resource was the budding mental health industry 55 years ago. This was the only resource used that "I actually saw or heard." My parents deeply regretted using these methods. It only made me worse. I was "studied," not changed or helped in any way. I am very happy for kids now who can receive better developed help from this industry and that more Christians are trained professionals in it.

After a "cutting episode and disappearing episodes", I ended up being in three mental hospitals as an inpatient. My parents (imperfect as we all are) were absolutely **desperate** to help me. At that time the mental health industry was merely developing. They just sedated me, and I was given poor "Sigmund Freud" type counseling, including **sixteen** electric shock treatments. I was housed with adults. Presently, in the more advanced mental health industry, there is a different, less radical approach with children who are like I was. Also, children are not housed with adults. Practical and methodical "behavior modification" is used and it works and has been well developed over the years. But, various people were often wounded terribly in the long years of process during the "swaggering over- confidence" by doctors, newly developed labels and therapy, and eventually discards of it all! They finally have more **accurate and effective** mental health therapy and have landed in much better places.

Over these years, the industry has discovered that there are a significant number of kids who have specific traits and quirks in common. These traits are difficult to live with and can lead to a very poor life if not modified and /or corrected. Behavior modification and sometimes a light medication are used to reduce obsessive/ compulsive traits. Eye contact is poor in these children. Rare are the severe approaches used like my own treatment 50 years ago. This only caused more damage to me and great pain to my parents.

About seven years ago after a speaking luncheon where I was keynote speaker, several luncheon ladies approached me. They told me to look a particular diagnosis up. These traits that I had mentioned in detail in my testimony at the luncheon were exactly like the traits in their grandchildren who were being treated properly and fitting in better. *Very reluctantly*, I searched the Internet. I studied the dozen personality quirks on the Internet mental health sites, those traits that affected me long ago, and I **matched up to every single one.** The hair on the back of my neck stood up when I read them! I refrain from using a "label" as I was never diagnosed professionally. I refrain from those labels also out of fear that someone suffering from these traits would be offended by a mere lay person's self- diagnosis in hindsight. *A diagnosis is no longer important to me at all!*

*I even ended up at age 15 in a penal institution for a year.. totally evil and brutal. This was hidden from my hometown and my siblings. When I returned at age 16 I needed help over this brutality, but was told that I would be sent back if I uttered one word about it. I left the reform school with a deep nicotine habit and sexual identity problems and habits. Had I not surrendered my heart and life to God at age 22, I would imagine that is where I would be today, or dead in the woods somewhere.*

Hitchhiking one dark night, at age 22, on my way to New Orleans from South Carolina……. I reached out to Jesus Christ. This was as the result of my sister in law shyly giving me prophecies to study which lent to me **great evidence that Jesus must be real, instead of a myth. God knew that I was on a death march on that road. I had zero self-worth and chanced many dangerous risks with no thought, as was common with this condition.** I was only thinking how and when I would get to NOLA. I intended to be homeless there and a street person. SUDDENLY, I THOUGHT ABOUT THOSE PROPHECIES Susan had told me about. COULD JESUS BE REAL? SUDDENLY, OUT OF NOWHERE…. I REMEMBERED a sermon I heard 11 years earlier… **at age 10. (I don't remember last weeks' sermon!!)** The sermon was about the mustard seed. Jesus said we only have to have enough faith the size of a tiny mustard seed. It lit up my head because I felt that I had at least the faith of a tiny mustard seed now, with the evidence from the prophecies that had been fulfilled in the Middle East. But I was so worthless, with many evil habits, quirks and addictions and a generally "unlikable" personality. Suddenly, I also remembered a TV show I saw at home featuring the Billy Graham evangelist. I use to think how **hokey** it was that all those people went up to the alter while Billy Graham said "Come just as you are, Come just as you are"… let **God** change you." And so, with that final memory flooding my head on that dark highway, I had *permission* to go to God *just as I was!*

I prayed out loud on that pitch black highway while I walked. I said "Jesus, if you are real, I want you. *I want you.* I want you to change me into just an *ordinary* person." That was my simple prayer and *God knew I meant it.* I don't think that I glowed in the dark, but there was an overwhelming sense of something supernatural flooding my being. The big difference that surprised me was that I had **never been scared on a dark road hitchhiking**.... (because I had zero self-worth) . **Suddenly I was very afraid** of the woods, the cars, and the dark. **I realize in hindsight that I suddenly cared about myself and was filled with a new self-worth**. The difference was the gift of the Holy Spirit, given to me because I truly meant that prayer of surrender. Also, I had **never, ever changed my mind** in the past about disappearing, which was *one trademark of peculiarity* since childhood. I FELT STRENGTH IN MY SHOULDERS AS IF SOMEONE WAS HOLDING THEM.... AND I TURNED AROUND TO FACE THE DIRECTION HOME. A GREAT ACT OF COURAGE FOR ME..... TO FACE THE MUSIC WHEN I DID

NOT HAVE TO. A paperback New Testament had been given to me by my sister in law. She knew my limitations and realized that I would not be likely to read a more "sophisticated" version. The next morning I absorbed it. I believed it. God showed me practical application in His word and I DID IT!

Another supernatural thing happened. When I woke up the next morning everything in creation seemed a more vivid color. Everything and every feeling seemed new. It was strange. I have since learned that people who have death experiences and see Heaven almost always say that the colors were more vivid and bright. I had never read that at that time, but I was struck by it and not expecting it! I totally understand that the Spirit of God **does not rush upon and fill every believer** as it did me. *It is not a "fourth of July" experience for each believer.* It was never like that for my husband. But his faith was strong. **However quiet and sullen this Spirit is in your life and without** *dramatic manifestations,* He can still be the "whisperer" leading you to power, enthusiasm, and the right path. Do not feel "scandalized" by a quiet and sullen filling and direction of the Holy Spirit. We all need something different. God knows us! I am led now by His quiet and sullen whisperings and it is just as exciting as the beginning!

I was changed little by little over the next fifteen years and beyond that. I stopped medications and therapy. However, I know that in other believer's lives, they are very grateful when the Holy Spirit leads them to the right medication and the right Christian counselor! Our journeys are all unique and different!

Amazing how my marriage and kids and life turned out! After the kids were adults, my late life career as a Personal Trainer has been blessed for 23 years and I became a noted speaker, including health and fitness from God's perspective. I spoke as keynote speaker to Women's luncheons and God gave me the words.... Scared to death! I was not "zapped" of all peculiarities. It was a long process. I still have some. People either run to me, or away from me!! I am always surprised that a few people actually call me and want my company! I treasure friends! I am no longer a loner! In junior high I hid in bathroom stalls not able to be conversational with kids and avoiding bullies. In high school I went to the bleachers and smoked alone or stole from people's things in the gym. I never went to a football game or a prom. I have never been to a reunion.

My marriage turned out good and it lasted 30 years, growing together in Christ, until my husband died. The Lord *"broke each one of us in all the right places,"* and we never gave up on our holy sacrament of marriage, or making it enjoyable instead of miserable! My two kids are real "stand outs" in their marriages and in their careers and in their love walk with Christ. I recognized right away that they were not like me when they were just little. I actually learned some behavior modification *from them* when they were young....they were very sharp socially. My daughter still helps me gently and kindly when I regress on some small thing! My son and his children tell me if I am speaking too loudly, repeating myself, or interrupting. They love me as I am but I have improved greatly!

I LIVE AMAZED...... JUST AMAZED. **This life and how it turned out should not be true. John 10:10** says that "Satan comes to steal, kill, and destroy but Jesus Christ comes to give us life to the **full and abundant!**" I want everyone to know that the word of God and the entire "trinity" can make a huge difference... huge. **My personal <u>behavior modification</u> was** "addiction to behavior guidelines in sacred scripture and the difficult application" of it, and also the right husband for 30 years!!

Three months after the divine encounter with the Lord, we joined a church. My husband was raised Southern Baptist but had fallen away. *At that time*, this was the group that God wanted me to be part of and I followed my husband... and attended the Southern Baptist Church in each town that we lived in. I always wanted to shout from the rooftop the reality of Jesus Christ and the power of his Word. .

Some areas of change took longer than others, **such as the food addiction.** But God did not give up on me. I have so enjoyed the freedom and changes in this area of food addiction that had me in miserable bondage from age seven to age 45!

**God helped me to forget HOW to be food addicted!**

**A Favorite Memory Verse**

*I will ask the Father, and He will give you another Counselor to be with you forever. He is the Spirit of truth.*
**(John 14: 16-17 HCSB)**

I opened the Bible in 1972 in a lonely church parking lot and read for the first time about "our Counselor". There were actually three chapters explaining the meaning of "our Counselor." *These words hit me between the eyes.* Over the years my parents had paid handsomely for many mental health counselors. However, those counselors had not been able to stop me from destroying myself. I discovered on that night that I had a free mental health counselor at my disposal! He would lead me into *all truth* about myself and everything else in this world, just one step at a time through practical, relevant scriptures if I would just continue to turn to Him! (He has also led me with church, traditions, the saints here, and the awesome examples of the Saints in Heaven! Those folks have always motivated me!)

I was in the church parking lot alone that night, because that evening at home my husband and I had tempers that flared into a vicious and frightening argument. I desperately wanted to run from this nightmare. *I wanted to quit.* I drove to the empty church parking lot, feeling that I had no one to talk to but God. I had my Bible with me, as always. As a new Christian, I asked God to tell me what the reason was that I had *not* gone down to the corner bar to seek comfort drinking and talking to other men. What had kept me from that temptation or just running away and disappearing again? Here in this verse and in chapters 14, 15, and 16. I found the *reason* I was making different choices than in the past when upset and frantic. The Holy Spirit Himself *was inside me now* and had become my **primary Counselor**. *My Counselor, Helper, Comforter and Advocate (the Holy Spirit) is far more capable than any earthly medical man or woman or mind altering drug. He leads me into Truth. He will seldom tell me more Truth until I am practicing what I already have! He anchors me in practicing all truth, one step at a time!*

In 2016 I became a charismatic Catholic, joining in the lifelong worship experience of my daughter in law's family (she and the family are the most Christ centered people I have EVER known.)

All Christian churches, Protestant and Catholic, have guidelines about "when" and "how" we truly receive this amazing Holy Spirit. **Father Cedric Pisegna** is an on fire, passionate "Priest Evangelist", welcomed by Protestants and Catholics, (often on TBN and Daystar) and he says it well. It is not a direct quote from him but he said something like *"God can break these rules. He knows when to flood someone with the Holy Spirit and change their lives! God is not regulated nor confined with the guidelines of any church doctrines to come and live within a person. God is far bigger than that!!"*

Most of us learn deeply and significantly from *our own personal journey* with God. God speaks to each of us in a unique way, sometimes through sermons or a Godly person or an inspirational book. Sometimes through the many bible readings from church. But when He speaks to us in our "closet, quite time" through sacred scripture passages, each of us knows when it is a *word meant for us.* It is **straight** from the supernatural Trinity and no other earthly person. It touches our hearts and impacts us as though it was God Himself speaking directly to us, to help us with the *very situation* we are in.

Prayer is talking to God. Reading and running to God's word is Him talking to you. *Sometimes we listen!*

### <u>MY FAVORITE MEMORY VERSE</u>

*For the word of God is living and active, sharper than any two edged sword, piercing to the division of soul and spirit, of joints and marrow, and discerning the thoughts and intentions of the heart.*

Hebrews 4:12 RSV)

When I saw this verse in 1972, it totally described what I felt like when I began reading the little Good News Bible, the day after my conversion. When we truly surrender our lives to Christ, the Holy Spirit fills us with desire to read God's Word, with power to pray, and with courage to share his Word with others. THE WORD WAS ALIVE. It had never taken on life before! Or at least, I had never

## My First Memory Verse

*Consider it pure joy, my brothers, whenever you face trials of many kinds, because you know that the testing of your faith develops perseverance. Perseverance must finish its work, so that you may be mature and complete, not lacking anything.*
**(James 1: 2-4 NIV)**

The day right after my dramatic conversion experience at age twenty-two, I quickly read through the little paperback version of the New Testament which was paraphrased in the ordinary language of everyday speech. You might say I devoured the words before my eyes. It was a true awakening to *God's willingness to speak to me.*

As I moved through that little volume hungrily, I came upon this verse about perseverance. *I made many important realizations. I understood right away that I would need change in my behavior. Not just a small change, but lots of it, and in many areas. I realized that the work I needed to do would not happen overnight. It would take a big decision, and plenty of time and effort.*

For a young person who had been hospitalized repeatedly for mental disorders, changing even a few of my dysfunctional, anti- social behaviors seemed a tall order. The words of this passage weren't the *least bit appealing* to me! It was a mandate for **challenging repentance – a growth process which would clearly take unpleasant effort and patience**. But with this realization, the Lord had begun His slow and kind process of helping me to become more like Himself. With His help, I had a brand new hope that I could be "ordinary" and I would gradually develop a harvest of good things in my life, instead of experiencing a long life of the same negative patterns and the difficult consequences they brought with them.

This first brush with the Holy Scripture speaking to me very personally turned into a *lifetime love relationship* of ***"letting God write His story into my own."***

For 20 years I practiced evangelism with a platform of various prison ministries. For 15 years I practiced evangelism with a platform of health/fitness ministries as motivational speaker and author. God gave me courage though I felt not qualified. God does not always call the qualified… sometime He calls us first and makes us qualified!

At age sixty one, *after accumulation of five small grandchildren* and pouring myself into them, I practiced evangelism only as a small group leader in bible and prayer study leading a non-denominational group. Four Protestants and three Catholics. This was a small, quiet, and non-descript ministry, which was a favorite for five years, filled with sweet blessings at the feet of Jesus, with no titles, and strong interactions of the Holy Spirit for the ladies. It further amazes me that age 69 and with grandchildren whom I spend lots of time with, that I am still **gripped** with wanting *unbelievers* in Christ to know the truth and wanting *believers* to be stronger.

From age 58-61 I was with a large women's club as a luncheon speaker trained with an evangelical address, asking for their decisions to surrender to Christ. My first book in print was approved by the large women's group for book tables. I am not a writer, but God intervened with amazing help to give me great writers to help me. The Writer's Guild even asked me to be guest *speaker **twice!!*** I appreciate the people with a true strong writer's gift. Some of us just have a message that needs to be written and it was a divine intervention the books were recognized by **anyone at all!**

The women's group was non-denominational with many Catholics attending, but a substantial number of fundamentalist evangelicals at its core, including me, before I changed to Catholicism. Among the 1200 groups in the nation, numerous Catholics served as chair women. These Catholic women were obviously gripped as I was for unbelievers in Christ. Their love and tolerance of some people in the group who criticized their Catholic traditions was always a striking example of love for me. Love is powerful. They consider Protestants their "brothers and sisters in Christ." All Protestants should also *recognize* the similarities that we have: the Virgin Birth, the Crucifixion, the Resurrection, the Ascension, the focus of the Holy Spirit and our common enemy – Satan. We have this in common. That does not mean we must leave our own faith groups, but this should be recognized by Protestants! I pray that I can help build a bridge between us that only love can build, instead of the continual hateful and snide remarks I heard privately from some Protestants, in all faith groups, in regard to differences. That broke my heart and is still a knife in my heart. (I was an evangelical Protestant and so people felt free to comment like this in front of me). They do not have to agree with all tradition and theology that Catholics hold so very dear, but they should say just as the Catholics say, "that we are their brothers and sisters in Christ," and just **stop right there**, short of the rants and criticisms. That Crucifix represents the suffering of Christ and how he paid the price for our sins with his blood. He suffered for us... He loved us.... We can suffer for Him and *do it well* as we look at that Crucifix. I was also very excited in my new evangelical Catholicism when we celebrated the Resurrection for **50 whole days after Easter!** That was new and amazing to me, but so I was saddened by the *myth* that we don't celebrate Resurrection, just Crucifixion. So sad at all the myths I had believed myself with no research, just primarily by conjecture and the passing down of missconceptions.

For the last 14 years, my main focus has been to be a strong witness to my **FIVE Catholic grandchildren**. Their family loves sacred scripture, very charismatic and *filled* with the Holy Spirit, and we bond perfectly. I am praying over new evangelism platforms as I will have more time. My son's family large extended family through marriage "loved me into Catholicism at age 66!" Also, some very Christ centered

Catholic personal training clients did the same thing. Not a word from any of them in regard to conversion ---- they just LIVED their faith with astounding love and always had Jesus on their lips. I love my new faith just as I did my encounter with Christ 47 years ago. It has **"set me on fire"** once again! **I have finally found that comfort level that I never had. Right in the first church that Jesus started 2000 years ago. I find fault with plenty... (flawed people are in every church, including myself.... People who grow and learn.... But I can deal comfortably with it where I am now and be able to focus on many great things.)**

God truly made me *ordinary,* just as I asked Him to do on my dark highway prayer. I blend in more with people to be of some "earthly good." My "heavenly good" makes me a little different than our world as most people see it, but God says that a Christian is "called to be different." God is my new husband and my twenty foot Pontoon on a boat slip is my boyfriend! That is certainly different but it gives me peace and keeps my good habits and protects my purity in my walk with the Lord! The front of my boat is detailed with "My Floating Boyfriend." People get a kick out of it! God kept me in my faith all through the years with many, many challenges. Some of my challenges were my husband's long illness and death, early serious marital problems, problems with teenagers, financial problems, and addictions including bondage to obesity. The loneliness as a widow in my fifties and the kids gone at the same time was the most difficult and where I really fell hard and long for five years. Early on in my twenties and thirties, I also always felt the shame of being very different, with some *lingering peculiarities*, which was a sad challenge at times, which God always overcame. I am not weird, but unique! YAY!! **11 Corinthians 12: 8-9** says that God's power shows up best in our weakness.

He has given me courage to fight injustice on many levels with God's courage. I fought the KKK one time when all others ran and were silent! I fought to integrate my Southern Baptist church in 1973 in Florida. I had two African American friends who attended with me and I was so naïve until a "meeting" was called to keep them from coming! At first the people hated me, but then the Holy Spirit took over and convicted them with love.

It is never, ever easy. Satan is un-relenting. <u>**1 Peter 5: 8**</u> says "our adversary roams the earth like a hungry lion, looking for a victim to tear apart. Resist him and in a short while God will lift you up and put you on high ground." <u>**1 John 4:4**</u> says "He that is in us, is greater than he who is in the world." If we **step out** for righteousness in Christ Jesus, we need these profound scriptures and contemplative, specific prayer as the Bible and the Catechism teaches.

### <u>A favorite verse.</u>

> <u>*Christian Apologetics who give us rational reasons to believe*</u> *Study thyself approved unto God, a workman that needeth not to be ashamed, rightly dividing the word of truth.*
> 
> **II Timothy 2:15 KJ)**

This verse impresses me because I discovered very early on that to express God's truth, I had to study, study, study as this scripture says, and I had to practice at expressing that truth. This is why I keep my memory scriptures printed out together so that I can review them and not lose them. I became a believer as a result of study and searching for evidence. Forty four years later I still enjoy reading scholars of apologetics, who provide **rational reasons** to embrace the faith and the word of God as infallible. There is no part that is accidental or unnecessary! The fact that it took fifteen hundred years to canonize and was written by over forty authors is *just more* evidence to these scholars of its total truth. Some of my favorite apologetic scholars are as follows:

**Lee Strobel** wrote **"The Case for Christ"** and traveled the world to prove that Christianity was only a myth. In the process he became a believer! It contains overwhelming scientific and historical evidence that defies probability. **Scott Hahn,** former Protestant, has studied Catholic history from the day that Christ ascended and the church was established. He presents a moving case to help with all the myths that have been handed down since the Reformation. All documented. My favorite document is the "description of worship 100 AD, which is a perfect description of our Mass!! **Josh McDowell** is one of my favorites. His book **Evidence That Demands a Verdict** is outstanding and proves biblical prophecy. **C.S. Lewis**, the renowned British college professor began his career as an **atheist**. After reading the Bible, he received the gift of faith, converted, and wrote **Mere Christianity** which has inspired many. Though he never had full conversion to Catholicism, this book brought many Catholics to full surrender to faith in Christ and they came home to

Catholicism. It is considered by many to still be the best book to bring an atheist to conversion to Christianity. It has also brought many Evangelicals to Catholicism. **Dr. Carl Baugh** addresses the issue of the evolution of man from higher mammals. He is one of thousands of scientists who spend their lives producing solid scientific evidence that evolution is at best a theory, at worst a hoax. Historian **David Barton** collected a stunning amount of written historical evidence that America was built upon the gospel. He wished to build the case for our Biblical foundations, to disprove the lies which have flourished in modern times.

These apologetics know how to address the doubts of this world and they present ten times more hard evidence than their opponents do. They study constantly just as my memory scripture instructs, and can debate down to the core the issues of the day that lead people away from God's truth. In my opinion, the atheistic scholars use very little hard evidence in comparison to these believing scholars. People who simply don't want to obey a loving God do not demand much evidence. **Joseph Greenfield, the attorney and professor who started the Harvard Law School,** claims that in a courtroom he would have excessive hard evidence from historical documents to convict Jesus Christ as having risen from the dead. For example, it is documented in history that **Saint Claudia,** (the wife of Pontius Pilate) saw Jesus ascended and she lived underground as a Christian and was martyred. Why would she abandon riches and status as the Roman governor's wife to be hunted, tortured and killed for her beliefs? Well, she saw Jesus murdered and buried and she saw him **raised from**

**the dead.** She had no choice but to believe! ALL of the disciples were fearful and hiding and denying Christ during and after the crucifixion of our Lord. Why did ALL of these same fearful men later choose to live for Christ and die for Him? They **saw him resurrected and were filled with the Holy Spirit** later, who gave them courage to live for Him until they were martyred.

Google and study these apologetics among dozens of others and at *the very least* stop saying that believers have fallen into a hole of ignorance or have a pathetic need. Our faith is based upon evidence which **defies the scientific law of probability.**

*Blind faith is not necessary. However, the last and most important step is childlike faith.*

**1 Corinthians 13....** The entire chapter declares the power and importance of Love. I love my brothers and sisters in Christ. *We need each other more than ever!* Can we be brothers and sisters in Christ with kind and gentle words only?

If we die for Him, will it be hand in hand *together* focusing on the death and resurrection of our Savior as we face our own eternity and talk to God face to face? When we are with others who worship Christ differently, can we just focus on being **kind?** Can we just be glad that others have discovered Christ as Lee Stroeble and C.S. Lewis did?

How can atheists embrace our faith if those who profess that Jesus is God argue hatefully?

## IN CLOSING:

Paul was an evangelist, reaching over the world to unbelievers, sharing his Damascus Road experience on his own dark highway. Paul speaks to Timothy who he mentors and Paul knows that his time to be alive is short. **2 timothy 4:5:** "Timothy, keep your head in all situations, and endure hardship and do the work of an evangelist, discharging all the duties of your ministry."

In our modern day, our brothers and sisters in Christ, all over the world are dying for their faith in Jesus. In America, we often think to ourselves that God **would give us the courage to die for him.** But the real question is for us, for all American Protestants and Catholics is:

**Will we <u>LIVE</u> for Him????** In our modern day, with cultural changes, it is very hard to LIVE for Christ and then take a courageous, but loving stand.

A quote from Jonathan Edwards, Patriot 1700's

"Number one: I will live for Christ."

"Number two: I will live for Him if no one else does!"

*"Always be prepared to give an answer to everyone who asks you to give the reason for hope that you have, but do this with gentleness and respect".*
**1 Peter 3:15 NIV**

*"I have competed well; I have finished the race; I have kept the faith."*
**11 Timothy 4:7 NAB**

(Paul says this with relief and amazement of all that God has completed in his life. He awaits execution. (Many translations say "I have fought the good fight", which I hope I will say!)

**1 John 4:2 HCSB** Every Spirit who confesses that Jesus Christ has come in the flesh is from God. But every spirit who does not confess Jesus is not from God." (We all have our differences, but according to that scripture this is the main way to know counterfeit Christianity.) "Counterfeit Christian experts" (a large Internet group) go way beyond this clear scripture and it is very hateful and *not confined* to anti-Catholicism. Their hate is camouflaged with a feeling of good intention to protect "real" Christians and "correct theology" from counterfeit Christians. Many groups are attacked. I even heard Billy Graham included in an attack! It is so sad that I cry and shake my *head*.

*I love all my brothers and sisters who claim that no one but Jesus is God. It is a bold and* **courageous** *claim in this world! And I know that God is madly in love with those who don't believe in Christ and he wants us to tell them the Good News, but with love!*

We have our differences in how to worship in certain areas, but we will all be together one day! We focus on Jesus Christ and the Holy Spirit and telling the Gospel story to all but with respect and gentleness.

**Ephesians 4:32 HCSB** "Be **kind and compassionate** to one another, forgiving one another, just as God in Christ Jesus also forgave you."

# Appendix

*A brief list of more structured help for you in the form of websites and books.*

<u>Bariatric Foodie... Foodie Nation</u> **THIS IS A MUST! The best blogging site on the Internet to encourage patients with the truth** about their surgery and a lot of nutritional help specific to surgery restrictions and healthy, hearty, fun recipes. Great vitamins and foods for sale! Great guidance from Nikki in regard to struggles. Great referrals to Bariatric experts. Great discussions to encourage each other! www.bariatricfoodie.com

<u>**Tracking Your Exercise Minutes and your Calorie Boundaries with Cell Phones**</u>**:**

www.Myfitnesspal.com is one among many. Another favorite is www.livestrong.com Find one that is user friendly to you. This will be a lifelong habit. I still track after 23 years. **Now, the tracking is easy and extremely educational just from doing it!** Almost all of these are managed by people who have very academic degrees in food and exercise. Make sure it is headed by a Registered Dietician and Exercise Physiologists. Stay away from the typical diet doctor if they have a site. There is a chance they will teach you the same old starvation they have practiced for years, and they fully believe in this despite the facts and clinical long-term results that we see all around us.

<u>WEBSITE</u>: www.Choosemyplate.gov

This site is by the United States Department of Agriculture. There is no bias and no ulterior motive financially. All of my resources basically agree with the science reflected in this site. This is much improved over the old Food Pyramid. But I think it was a surprise to many who waited on the changes that protein and fat was not listed as the major portion of good diets. The body has not changed!

**BOOK:** *Made to Crave,* by Lysa Terkeurst. (Zondervan, December 15, 2010)

I love the way she describes **entering weight maintenance** as the "danger zone." So right!

**BOOK**: *Small Changes, Big Results,* by Ellie Krieger. (Clarkson Potter, Feb 22, 2005)

Ellie gives very structured help with food and exercise, which I realize some people's *personality profiles* need. She also includes the importance of changing the mind and being aware of lifestyle issues. She is a Registered Dietician, which is all that I listen to, after years of fast weight loss doctors failing me.

<u>**GROUP**</u>: Weight Watchers

*Too much structure did not fall into line with my personality* profile. Weight Watchers was good for me because it allows you to have anything to eat that you want within the "point range," while still stressing good clinical nutrition. This is under the umbrella of Registered Dieticians. They also address lifestyle issues and the mind in their entertaining lectures. (For me, I just kept up with calorie boundaries, which in my opinion must be 75% of the point concept). *Weightwatchers.com You will of course be deleting and changing foods based upon your surgery.*

**GROUP:** Celebration Recovery Program, by Rick Warren. Google it. For all types of addictions.

**WEBSITE:** www.weightlossresources.co.uk/diet/dietitian.htm

**Juliette Kellow, Registered Dietician**. Excellent academics presented to keep you motivated with all truth.

**BOOK:** Dr. Howard Shapiro's Picture Perfect Weight Loss Book, (Grand Central, 2003)

He is a doctor, but not a fast weight loss doctor! He illustrates in beautiful color pictures of meals and treats which satisfy, satiate, and don't deprive. He has the calories on the pictures, and shows comparisons of how much more volume you can have when you make better choices. Everyone should have these illustrations on their book shelf. Food should be a friend, not an enemy!

**TRAINERS:** Apex Fitness. Apex trainers are among the minority of trainers who actually have a nutrition certification under the umbrella of Registered Dieticians. The mentality is the same as Weight Watchers. No forbidden foods and a wide of variety of foods and the calorie boundaries are stressed.

Supplements are promoted but not frivolous ones. ("Search the site" to find a trainer in your area) www.apex-fitness.com

**TRAINERS:** Anytime Fitness gyms. Find a freelance (self-employed) trainer, who might have more leverage in helping you and are often more affordable than trainers in large athletic clubs.

**BOOK**: *Sports Nutrition Guidebook*, by Nancy Clark, MS, RD (Human Kinetics, May 2008)

**TRAINERS:** www.acefitness.org (fitness information and great trainer locator)

# NOTES

Scripture verses are from the NIV (New International) New American Bible, Revised King James, and the King James Bible.

Author Dr. Charles Swindoll. Source from internet devotions. "A Very Present Help".

Chuck Swindoll www.insight.org

Oswald Chambers, book "My Utmost for His Highest"... edited by James Reimann... Date 1992 Discovery House Publishers

Author Dr. Charles Stanley. The devotion "The Ultimate Race". In Touch Magazine, December 2006.

Apex Fitness Manuel. The quote "the greatest amount of calories with the least amount of exercise." Fitness Manuals and seminars: quotes in regard to "we use to run after our food"......... Apex Fitness Manuals. The quote "gym science verses real science."

The Dreaded Plateau.... Paraphrased from the Manuel.

The quotes under myths in regard to "carbs, fat, and protein make us fat. Wrong! Too many calories make us fat", etc. This is paraphrased from their manual. Paraphrases and comments from me in interpretation of Neal Spruce's chapter on genetics.

Primary author of Apex Training Manual is Neal Spruce, copyright 2004.

The term "Skill Power, Not Will Power" comes from The Balancing Act, by Georgia Kostas, MPH, RD Published by The Balancing Act, October 1998

The phrase "the strength of the surgery alone" is borrowed from bariatriceating.com. (rants)

CPSIA information can be obtained
at www.ICGtesting.com
Printed in the USA
LVHW110903100722
723141LV00005B/98